SIMON DOBSON

EPIDEMIC MODELLING – SOME NOTES, MATHS, AND CODE

Contents

To everyone trying to understand, control, or treat epidemic disease.
The job will never end. That's what makes it essential.

Acknowledgements

Thanks to the students and collaborators who have helped me to get more and more interested in complex networks over the years, and whose knowledge and enthusiasm have been so motivating: Davide Cellai, Xue Guo, Peter Mann, John Mitchell, Stefan Nixon, Martynas Noreika, Aleksejs Sazonovs, Saray Shai, Anne Smith, Mike Pitcher. The fact that I still understand so poorly remains my fault.

Thanks to the friends and colleagues who asked about epidemic modelling and were then sucked into commenting, proof-reading, and listening to half-formed explanations: Diego Arenas Contreras, Muffy Calder, Simone Conte, Lisa Dow, Lei Fang, Ian Gent, Fenella Hayes, Julie McCann, Conor Muldoon, Riccardo Romano, Juan Ye. No good deed goes unpunished.

Thanks to the University of St Andrews for providing both a stimulating academic home and access to the computing resources needed to crunch the numbers.

This book would not exist without covid-19. Whether that is something to thank it for, or something further to blame it for, I leave up to you.

Preface

We've unexpectedly found ourselves in a situation in which
the science of diseases is of critical importance to us all. On an
individual level, we want to know what to expect of lockdowns,
vaccines or other therapies. At a population level, we want to
know how diseases become epidemics and then pandemics, and
how the different strategies might influence their course. Above
all, we want certainty that the disease will be conquered and the
future will be better.

Scientists don't really *do* certainty, though. All of science is
based around the *models* that we construct to tell us about the
things we're interested in, and the *experiments* that we conduct
to see whether the models match the reality on the ground. It's
this combination of model and experiment, trial and error and
correction, that help us understand the world.

But what *is* a model of a disease? How do they work, and what
can they tell us about what we can expect from epidemics and
other events? I'm writing this book as an attempt to explain the
one small corner of this vast field that I know something about:
how to model epidemics using network science and computer
simulations. It isn't in any way comprehensive, leaving huge
areas unexplored and a huge number of questions unanswered. I
make it available as a work in progress in the hope that it may be
useful and may encourage an interest in science.

Models and modelling

We should first clarify what is means to model something, or to develop a model: what models are, what we expect from them, their advantages and limitations.

Models

By **model** we mean a formal description of some aspects of a system of interest that we can explore in order to gain insight into the behaviour of the real system.

A **mathematical model** consists of one or more equations expressing the relationships between different quantities. There are often some **parameters** involved, quantities whose values are known or assumed.

A **computational model**, by contrast, is a program written to simulate the behaviour of the system. Such simulations are almost always based on underlying mathematical models and include parameters. What do computers provide? Sets of equations can often be understood (or "solved analytically") by purely symbolic means, but many systems of equations *can't* be solved this way and instead need to be solved numerically, by starting with specific values (numbers) and showing how they evolve under the equations. Even for equations that *can* be solved analytically, computers are often useful tools for helping to explore large systems, or for visualising the results.

One can also have **mechanical** models, of course, such as the orreries that model the motions of planets. In some senses machines are just computation models that happen to use analogue components rather than digital.

Uses of models

There are lots of questions we might want to ask about systems, and these can often give rise to different models drawing on different styles and approaches to modelling. For definiteness, let's discuss some of the questions we might ask about epidemics.

We might be interested in **epidemics in general**. How do changes in infectiousness affect the spread of the disease? What are the relationships between infectiousness and recovery? How do different patterns of contacts in a population affect how it spreads? What are the effects of different countermeasures, like physical distancing, vaccination, or quarantine? Are there any patterns in the epidemic, like multiple waves? These are quite abstract questions that could be asked of *any* disease, and answering them might tell us something about how *all* diseases behave – including those we encountered yet.

On the other hand, we might be interested in **a specific disease**, or even in **a specific outbreak**. How will *this* disease spread in a population? How about in another country to the one it's currently in? How will a *particular* countermeasure affect the spread? When will it be safe for the majority of people to return to work? These are all very concrete questions that depend on the exact details of the situation about which they're asked, and answering them may be massively useful in managing this situation. (Taylor provides an accessible discussion of the uses and interpretations of the well-known Imperial College model of covid-19's impact on UK NHS bed availability during the 2020 outbreak [1].)

[1] Paul Taylor. Susceptible, infectious, recovered. *London Review of Books*, 42(9), May 2020

There's a saying among doctors who deal with outbreaks on the ground: "When you've seen one pandemic, you've … seen one pandemic." The lessons learned often don't translate to new situations.

The interplay between these two kinds of questions is quite complicated. In concrete cases we presumably measure the specifics of the outbreak and work with them. We only have partial control, for example on enforcing social distancing. It's often hard to then make more general predictions about diseases more widely, to draw conclusions that can be used in other cases.

Models and modelling

So should we be more abstract? Abstraction typically brings control over the model: we can explore a whole range of modes of transmission, for example rather than just the one we happen to have for this disease. We can explore different countermeasures in the model without committing to one, which means there are no consequences for being wrong. We get to observe some general patterns and draw general conclusions – which then don't *exactly* apply to *any* real disease.

On the other hand, the conclusions we draw from these abstract models can't be applied blindly to particular situations on the ground. A good example (which we'll come to later) concerns the conditions under which an epidemic can get established in a population. One would want to be *very* careful in taking the results of an abstract investigation of this phenomenon and then concluding that an epidemic can't occur in a specific population – very careful that the model's assumptions were respected, very careful that the parameters were known, and so forth. Mistakes in situations like this can mean that outbreaks get out of control, and people may die.

Assumptions

The accuracy of a model depends on its **assumptions**, and how well these match reality. This issue appears in several guises. The model's "mechanics" – the ways it fits its various elements together – need to match the disease it's (purporting to be) a model of. It needs to identify the parameters that control its evolution. These parameters need to match those of the real disease.

All these are problematic at the best of times, but especially when dealing with a new disease that's not been well-studied. How infectious is a disease? How long is a person sick for? Does the disease confer immunity on an individual who's had it? – and is that immunity total or partial, permanent or time-limited? All these factors introduce uncertainties into any conclusions we draw from modelling.

Correctness

Whether we're interested in concrete or abstract questions, we still have the problem of **correctness**: does our model produce the "right" answers? It might not, either because it has been built incorrectly (has "bugs" in computer terms – but mathematical equations have them too), or because we don't know the values of some of the parameters (especially problematic in the middle of an outbreak, when measurement often takes a back seat to treatment), or because there are aspects of the real world that we haven't considered but that affect the result (often the case for more abstract models).

We know quite a lot about building software, much of which applies to the building of computer models: unit testing, integration testing, clear documentation, source version control, and so on. With modelling we then face the additional problem of deciding whether the code we've built is fit for purpose.

Deciding what "fit" means is an interesting question in its own right. It's something we may only know retrospectively: did the results that came out of the model match what happened on the ground? We may not be able to measure exactly what *did* happen on the ground: did we count all the fatalities, or were some missed, or mis-diagnosed? For a more abstract model, how happy are we that our simplifications don't entirely divorce us from reality?

Computer scientists often split the question of assuring correctness into two parts: **verification** ("did we build the thing right?") and **validation** ("did we build the right thing?").

Stochastic processes

There's another problem.

Suppose you have the misfortune of becoming ill. For a fortnight you are infectious, and there's a chance that you'll infect anyone you meet. Now we know that you don't infect *everyone* – no disease (fortunately) is so contagious – so you infect a fraction of all those you *could* have infected. We can't usually predict this exactly, but the exact details may matter: rather than infect Aunt

Carol, who's a noted recluse who has no further opportunities to infect anyone else, you instead happen to infect Cousin Charlotte who's a noted party animal and goes on to spread the illness widely. So even if we know the general pattern of a disease, the exact way in spreads is affected by chance factors.

A system like this is referred to as a **stochastic process**. They include an element of randomness in their very nature: it's *not* a bug, it's a feature.

Now consider what this means for modelling. We can take exactly the same situation – the same disease, the same population – run the model twice, get two different answers – and them *both* be right! The way to think about this is that each run is a "possible outcome" of the disease. There may be several possible outcomes, and they may all be similar – or there may be radical differences. (We'll see an example of this in a later chapter.)

One way to think about what's happening is that each run of the model is sampling the distribution of possible outcomes. You expect to seldom see "unlikely" outcomes and mainly see "likely" ones – but sometimes you'll see an "unlikely" outcome by chance.

We often think that every problem has a "right" answer, but for stochastic processes this isn't the case: there are many "right" answers. It's attractive to think that we can simply "debug" our way out of trouble, but in fact we can't. There may be randomness we can't engineer away.

What to do? Actually, computer science is unusual in "normally" having single answers. If you ask a biologist how long butterflies live for, you don't expect her to go out and observed the lifespan of *every single butterfly* before answering. Instead you get a statistical answer: an average and some variance. It's the same for stochastic processes (or models): we run the model several times (possibly hundreds of times) for the same inputs, and collate the results.

At least in principle. It can be tricky to accomplish in practice, not least because computer scientists have expended a lot of ingenuity in making their pseudo-random number sequences less pseudo and more random.

In a computer model, it's often possible to actually reproduce exactly even a stochastic process, because the "random numbers" we use are actually only pseudo-random and so can be re-created. That can help in the narrow sense of seeing whether the model produces the same results given the same inputs *and* the same "random" numbers, but it doesn't help in the wider sense of capturing the behaviour of a system with *inherent* randomness.

Managing our expectations

This all sounds like modelling is a horrible mess. But the situation isn't hopeless. We just need to be careful.

The results we get from any model, of any kind, are tentative and suggestive and can generate insight into the system the model is seeking to represent, whether concretely or abstractly. There will always be factors outwith the model's consideration. The results aren't "true" in any exact sense. They need to be interpreted by people who understand both the phenomena *and* models *and* modelling. This will often lead to the realisation that the model needs to be changed, or extended or enriched, and sometimes even simplified and stripped-down, better to answer the questions that are being posed.

When we quipped in the preface that "scientists don't really do certainty", it's this that we had in mind.

This is captured by the classic aphorism, attributed to the statistician George Box, that "all models are wrong, but some are useful ... the approximate nature of the model must always be borne in mind".

> Science is sometimes criticised for pretending to explain everything, for thinking that it has an answer to every question. It's a curious accusation. As every researcher working in every laboratory throughout the world knows, doing science means coming up hard against the limits of your ignorance on a daily basis – the innumerable things that you don't know and can't do. This is quite different from claiming to know everything. ... But if we are certain of nothing, how can we possibly rely on what science tells us? The answer is simple. Science is not reliable because it provides certainty. It is reliable because it provides us with the best answers we have at present. Science is the most we know so far about the problems confronting us. It is precisely its openness, the fact that it constantly calls current knowledge into question, which guarantees that the answers it offers are the best so far available: if you find better answers, those new answers become science. ... The answers given by science are not reliable because they are definitive. They are reliable because they are not definitive. They are reliable because they are the best answers available today. And they are the best we have because

we don't consider them to be definitive, but see them as open to improvement. It's the awareness of our ignorance that gives science its reliability.

—Carlo Rovelli [2].

[2] Carlo Rovelli. *Reality is not what it seems: The journey to quantum gravity*. Penguin, 2017

Modelling, like experimentation, is both integral to science and subject to it: both a tool and an object of study, to be approached sceptically and refined through time. The study of epidemics is an excellent example of this process, and we can progressively refine our models better to reflect our improving understanding.

Questions for discussion

- What can models tell us about real-world disease epidemics?

- Suppose you were asked to advise political leaders on the basis of what a model predicts. Would you? What would you want them to know about the process of modelling?

Disease progression

Everyone suffers from a disease at some point. The lucky amongst us avoid anything more serious than influenza, measles, or (in my case, years ago) whooping cough. But all diseases share some common characteristics: characteristics so common, in fact, that their mathematical properties are shared by other processes that aren't actually diseases at all, including the spread of computer viruses [3] and the spread of rumours and other information.

The diseases in which we are interested are caused by *pathogens*, typically viruses or bacteria: simple living organisms that make their homes in humans (or other living organisms) and cause some adverse reaction as a result of their lifecycle. These pathogens can pass between individuals in a number of ways, causing the disease to spread. A disease might be **airborne**, able to live in the air and be breathed by passing individuals. It might be spread by **droplets**, coughed and sneezed into the environment or deposited on objects and picked up by future physical contact with the contaminated surfaces. Or it might be communicable only by **direct physical contact**, skin to skin, through sex, or a blood transfusion. It might be **foodborne**, transmitted through contaminated food that infects several people from a common source. It might be **vectored** through an animal, as is the case for malaria which has to be sporead by mosquitoes and can't spread person-to-person. Even diseases that don't *require* a vector may still incubate in animal hosts *as well* as in humans (this is suspected in the case of the

[3] Jeffrey Kephart and Steve White. Directed-graph epidemiological models of computer viruses. In *Proceedings of Research in Security and Privacy*, pages 343–359. IEEE Press, May 1991

Diseases that must be vectored through animals to infect humans are also known as **zoonoses**.

1918 "Spanish flu" pandemic [4]). And finally there is a class of **non-communicable** diseases such as cancer or heart disease, some of which are **hereditary**: not caused directly by pathogens but perhaps influenced by their presence, and perhaps made worse by infections.

[4] J.S. Oxford, A. Sefton, R. Jackson, W. Innes, R.S. Daniels, and N.P.A.S. Johnson. World War I may have allowed the emergence of the 'Spanish' influenza. *Lancet Infectious Diseases*, 2(2):111–114, February 2002

A disease becomes an **epidemic** when it infects a substantial fraction of a population within a short time. There's no universally accepted definition of how large a fraction is needed to classify an outbreak as an epidemic: for new or rare diseases even a small number of infections might be considered an epidemic, while some diseases persist in a population at a low level and then flare-up epidemically. If an epidemic infects people in several populations – typically several countries or several continents – than it is termed a **pandemic**.

Each different kind of disease will have its own characteristic **pathology**, how it affects the body of a person infected. It will also have its own **epidemiology** that controls how it spreads. Clinically, both these characteristics are extremely important; we will focus here on the epidemiology, but the pathology remains important because factors involved in how a disease progresses *in* individuals may have a profound effect on how it spreads *between* individuals.

Disease progression

A person's infection goes through several periods, starting with their **disease progression;infection**. Once infected, the disease resides **latent** in their system, developing its presence but not showing symptoms and not being infectious to others. After this latent period the disease becomes **infectious**, capable of being spread to others. Typically a person's infectiousness peaks and dies away before the end of the disease progression.

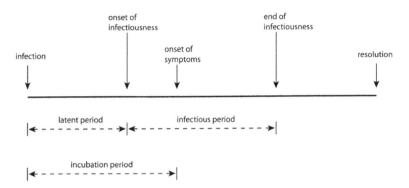

These two periods – latent and infectious – control the **transamission** of infection. After initial infection there will be an **disease progression;incubation period** before the person shows symptoms of the disease. After the onset of symptoms, the disease progresses and ends in some **disease progression;resolution**: the patient gets better, or dies. If they recover, they may then have some immunity to further infection.

For different diseases, the lengths of these periods and the ways they overlap vary. For **Type A** diseases, the incubation period is longer than the latent period. This means that a patient can start to transmit the disease before the disease becomes manifest in themselves. This happens in cases of measles and covid-19. In **Type B** diseases such as SARS or ebola, by contrast, the incubation period is shorter than the latent period, meaning that asymptomatic patients cannot infect others. So despite ebola being a more feared disease than measles, it may be easier to treat epidemiologically since quarantining patients showing symptoms will prevent transmission in the general population (although not to medical staff); in measles, transmission starts before symptoms show themselves, so quarantine based on symptoms is less effective. Moreover for some disease the infectious period may continue after the patient has died: the corpses of victims of ebola, which is transmitted *via* bodily fluids, can be extremely infectious for some time after death, meaning that funerals become very dangerous loci of potential infection for mourners.

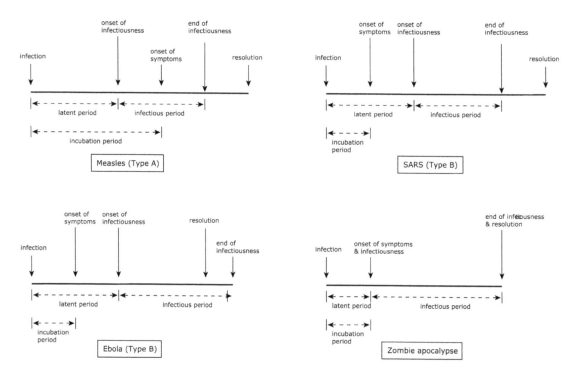

How long do the different periods last? For each disease there
will be typical durations, often with substantial variance. In the
case of ebola, for example, a typical timeline would be a 0–3 day
incubation period, a 7–12 day progression to recovery or death,
and a latent period of 2–5 days. The ranges give the variance of
periods, different for different individuals that depend on factors
including the severity of infection and the individual's overall
health. However, the incubation period for ebola can be up to
21 days, meaning that a suspected case needs to be quarantined
for this period: long enough, in other words, for the disease
symptoms to manifest if the person is actually infected. While
one can test for most diseases (including ebola) in a laboratory,
during an epidemic such tests may overwhelm the public health
infrastructure, making quarantine the most practical option.
(During historical disease outbreaks, of course, quarantine was
the *only* option.)

Measuring and modelling epidemics

Epidemiology is the science of creating models of diseases and their spread that can be analysed, to make predictions or to simulate the effects of different responses. To do this, we need to identify the core elements of a disease from the perspective of transmission: we typically do not need to understand the disease's detailed biology, only the timings and other factors that affect its spread.

We discussed above the periods of diseases, their relationships, and their different characteristics. We need some other numbers as well, however, and it turns out that these can be measured directly in the field.

The most important number is the **basic case reproduction number**, denoted $\mathcal{R}_0$. $\mathcal{R}_0$ represents the total number of secondary infections expected for each primary infection in a totally susceptible population. The 0 in $\mathcal{R}_0$ stands for $t = 0$: the basic case reproduction number applies at the start of an epidemic. Over the course of an epidemic the value of $\mathcal{R}$ will change as people become immune post-infection, countermeasures take effect, and so forth, and give rise to a **net case reproduction number** indicating how the disease is reproducing at a given time.

$\mathcal{R}$ is affected by three factors:

1. The **duration of infectiousness**. All other things being equal, a disease with a longer period of infectiousness has more time in which to infect other patients.

2. The **probability of transmission** at each contact. Some diseases are extremely contagious, with each contact having a high probability of passing on the infection; others are much harder to pass on to secondary cases.

3. The **rate of contact**. Someone coming into contact with a lot of susceptible individuals will have more opportunities to generate a secondary case than someone meeting fewer

people.

The first two factors are characteristic of the disease, derived from its biology. The third is characteristic of the social conditions in which the epidemic takes place: it is this factor that physical distancing, quarantine and so forth affect, by reducing (ideally to zero) the contacts an infected person has with uninfected individuals.

The importance of $\mathcal{R}$

The importance of $\mathcal{R}$ is that it indicates whether, and how fast, a disease can spread through a susceptible population. If $\mathcal{R} < 1$ then we expect fewer than one secondary case per primary. This means that each "generation" of the disease will be smaller than the one that infected it, and the disease will die out. If $\mathcal{R} = 1$ then the disease will perpetuate itself in whatever size of population was originally infected. Nature is never so precise as to present us with a disease like this, of course. However, $\mathcal{R} = 1$ is the **threshold value** at which diseases become epidemics. If $\mathcal{R} > 1$, the disease will break-out and infect more and more people exponentially quickly.

Exactly *how* quickly depends on how large $\mathcal{R}$ is. For measles, $\mathcal{R} \geq 15$ – fifteen new infections for each case – which explains how measles spread so quickly in unvaccinated populations. Different strains of influenza have different ranges of R: for the 1918 "Spanish flu" it has been estimated [5] that $1.2 \leq \mathcal{R} \leq 3.0$ in the community (although substantially more in confined settings). If this sounds benign, remember that this epidemic killed more people than the First World War. Perhaps interesting in light of its media coverage, for ebola we have $1.5 \leq \mathcal{R} \leq 2.7$ [6], roughly the same as a not-too-severe winter flu outbreak.

In a typical epidemic the number of people infected grows very quickly. If $\mathcal{R} = 2$ then one person infects two others, who each infect two others, who each ... and so on – so each generation is twice as big as the last). If you plot the size of the epidemic

[5] Emilia Vynnycky, Amy Trindall, and Punam Mangtani. Estimates of the reproduction numbers of Spanish influenza using morbidity data. *International Journal of Epidemiology*, 36:881–889, 2007

[6] Christian Althous. Estimating the reproduction number of Zaire ebolavirus (EBOV) during the 2014 outbreak in West Africa. *PLOS Currents Outbreaks*, September 2014

against time on a graph, it'll draw out an **exponential curve**.

Why we need to be careful about $\mathcal{R}$

This sounds like good news: if we know $\mathcal{R}$, we can estimate the size of the epidemic we're facing; if we calculate it on an on-going basis we can monitor how well any countermeasures we deploy are working, and decide when to relax those countermeasures.

Well, not quite. There are at least four reasons that mean we need to be careful not to over-rely on $\mathcal{R}$.

The first reason is mathematical. $\mathcal{R}$ is the exponent of the equation that controls the epidemic's size. This is important, because it means that epidemics behave **non-linearly**. An $\mathcal{R}$ value of 4 is not twice as bad as an $\mathcal{R}$ value of 2: the epidemic isn't twice as big, **it doubles twice as many times** in the same period. Small differences in the value of $\mathcal{R}$ therefore have huge effects.

This reason actually drives all the rest, because it acts as an amplifier for everything concerning $\mathcal{R}$.

It's true that $\mathcal{R} = 1$ is the critical value, below which an epidemic dies out. But it doesn't follow from this that an $\mathcal{R}$ value slightly over 1 is "pretty much 1" and so not a worry. **That non-linearity means that even a small excess in $\mathcal{R}$ can lead to a large outbreak**. This has implications for epidemic control too: reducing the $\mathcal{R}$ value to just below 1 isn't an indication that everything will then be fine, as a small increase may set things off again.

The second reason concerns estimation. The most effective way of estimating $\mathcal{R}$ is contact tracing, where infected individuals' contacts are located and tested – and can then be treated or isolated if found to be infected themselves. Careful and widespread "test, trace, and isolate" strategies can be extremely effective in reducing an epidemic. The number of infected contacts individuals have on average lets us estimate of $\mathcal{R}$.

But by definition **test and trace is "counting in the rear view**

Why we need to be careful about $\mathcal{R}$

mirror". It tells us how many people *were being* infected, not how many people *are being* infected. There will be a delay in identifying infected individuals, further delay in finding and testing their contacts, and so forth. If circumstances are changing, for example through pathogen evolution or it infecting different social settings, the estimate will be rendered out of date.

The third reason concerns the consequences of errors. **Finding, tracing, and counting of infected individuals is invariably error-prone**. People will be missed; tests are never 100% accurate, especially for diseases with long incubation periods where there may be low pathogen loads in the early stages; individuals forget whom they were in contact with; tracing apps don't work in all circumstances; and so forth. Each of these errors leads to under-counting secondary infections and therefore under-estimating R.

Finally we must remember that R is the *average* number of secondary cases per primary. The use of averaging (and indeed other summary statistics) is essential when trying to get the "big picture" of an epidemic. But it means that the value of R reported depends not just on the disease but on the population being averaged over.

To see what this might mean, consider a country consisting of one city surrounded by a collection of small villages – London in the Middle Ages might be a good example. Suppose the disease breaks out ferociously in the city but, because they are separated and take precautions, the villages see a much sparser rate of infection. If we were to compute the net case reproduction rate *averaged over the city* we'd capture all the ferocity of the epidemic's spread. But if we compute the rate *over the whole country*, we'd see a far milder epidemic. Because the same disease is spreading in different circumstances, averaging may be misleading – too mild for the city, but too large for the countryside. **When interpreting an average, you always need to know what population has been averaged over**. It is possible to manipulate the reported R value accidentally, or deliberately by judicious choice of population.

For all these reasons it's important not to fixate on $\mathcal{R}$. The fact that it's a number can sometimes give a false sense of security, because numbers suggest certainty and precision – and measuring $\mathcal{R}$ in the midst of an on-going epidemic offers neither. A value of $\mathcal{R}$ that's reducing over time is a good sign. But $\mathcal{R}$ falling – or *seeming* to fall – below 1 isn't enough to prove that countermeasures are working and can be relaxed.

Growth rates

You may have noticed that the definition of $\mathcal{R}$ doesn't include time. It's essentially the ratio of the different sizes of two "generations" of infection, and so tells us about the way the disease reproduces itself in a population. But it *doesn't* tell us *how fast* that reproduction happens: how long does it take for the "next generation" to come along?

Obviously the answer is something to do with the latent period we looked at earlier. The shorter the latent period, the faster an infected person becomes infectious, and the faster the epidemic will grow. $\mathcal{R}$ tells us nothing useful about this rate of growth.

Clearly this rate matters for tackling an outbreak, as well as for modelling the progress of a disease in time. For this reason it's common to use another, complementary measure of epidemic behaviour.

When we talked about the exponential growth in epidemic size, we were still thinking in terms of generations of disease. We can think in "real" time instead.

Mathematically, the size of an epidemic can be expressed as

$$N(t) \propto e^{\lambda t}$$

where $N(t)$ is the number of cases at time t (measured in some units) and λ is the **growth rate**, the number of new cases that appear per unit of time. The utility of this is that if we know the growth rate per day *and* we know how many disease cases we have *now*, we can predict how many diseases cases we'll have *later*, tomorrow (or even farther into the future) – and more importantly we'll know the answer in terms of days, not in terms of disease generations. Even more importantly, we can get λ directly from time series such as the number of diagnoses cases by **fitting** a theoretical curve to the collected data.

Just as $\mathcal{R}$ had a threshold at $\mathcal{R} = 1$ that determined whether the epidemic was growing or shrinking, so $\lambda = 0$ divides growing ($\lambda > 1$) from shrinking ($\lambda < 0$) conditions. And just like $\mathcal{R}$, we need to be careful about reading too much into that: mistakes or omissions in reporting the ongoing cases can easily cause an over- or under-estimate of λ.

A threshold value is an example of what mathematicians call a *seperatrix*, a value that divides two regimes of qualitatively different behaviour – growing or shrinking, in this case.

The values of $\mathcal{R}$ and λ are mathematically related, of course, with the former being found by integrating the latter [7]. In fact we can make λ capture just the biological part of the disease's spread, while capturing things like social issues and countermeasures separately as a probability distribution of infections over time.

[7] Jacco Wallinga and Marc Lipsitch. How generation intervals shape the relationship between growth rates and reproductive numbers. *Proceedings of the Royal Society B*, 274:599–604, 2007

Questions for discussion

- Think of a disease you've had. How did you catch it? Could you have done anything to *avoid* catching it? Was it made worse by where you lived at the time?

- What can be done to cope with "Type A" diseases, where people can transmit the disease without showing symptoms of it?

- Do you think the $\mathcal{R}$ number is a useful thing to keep track of during an epidemic? Why? (Or why not?)

Compartmented models

All disease models share some commonalities. Each model will need to represent the population of people being modelled, some (or all) of whom will get the disease in the course of the outbreak. It will need to represent the progress of the disease, as people are infected, become infectious, recover, and so forth. It will need some notion of how the disease spreads between people. And it will need to represent the disease dynamics: how long the various stages of the disease take, how virulently it spreads in the population, and so on.

There are many different ways to represent these phenomena, and each choice gives rise to a different modelling approach. There are a lot of trade-offs to be made, with more detail allowing more subtle issues to be captured and explored at the cost of making the model more complicated to understand and compute.

Let's start with what is perhaps the simplest model of an epidemic, the *SIR model*.

SIR: A compartmented model of disease

SIR is referred to as a *compartmented model* of disease. It represents the progress of the disease by specifying a number of states or *compartments*, with everyone in the population being assigned to exactly one compartment at anytime. The disease progresses by having people move between compartments according to some process.

SIR, as its name suggests, uses three compartments:

- **Susceptible (S)**, representing those people who can catch the disease;

- **Infected (I)**, representing those people who have caught the disease and can pass it on; and

- **Removed (R)**, representing those people whose infection has resolved itself and have been "removed" from progressing the disease any further.

Notice how simple this is. A person is either infected, or they're not. If they *are* infected, they are infectious: there's no latency. And they're "removed" when their infection resolves, without us noting whether they recovered or died.

You might ask whether something this simple can tell us anything: does any real disease work like this? But the simplicity of the model makes it tractable and easy to study, and once we've got a feel for how these things work we can, if desired, move onto more detailed models. SIR is just one of the possible compartmented models: the others include SIS (for diseases where you can be re-infected once recovered), MSEIR (for diseases with maternally-conferred temporary immunity), so so on in dizzying array (see Hethcote[8] for a more detailed discussion). We'll look at another model, SEIR, later.

[8] Herbert Hethcote. The mathematics of infectious diseases. *SIAM Review*, 42(4):599–653, December 2000

The mathematical model

We now need to describe how individuals move between compartments. Actually we'll simply talk about the *number* of people in each compartment at each time, and how those numbers change: we won't track the disease's progress in a specific individual (there's a whole class of *agent-based* models that do this).

Suppose we have a population of size N. Let's represent the number of people in each compartment by S, I, and R respectively. Everyone in the population is assigned to exactly one compartment at any time, so we must always have $S + I + R = N$ as the sub-populations S, I, and R change.

How does someone become infected? – that is to say, how does someone move between compartment S and compartment I? In SIR we assume that the infection passes through contact between a susceptible individual and an infected one. If we further assume that everyone in the population meets everyone else equally often, then there will be $S \times I = SI$ encounters between susceptible and infected individuals in each time period. Think of the population as crowd milling around, some of whom are infected.

Clearly not all of these interactions will result in an infection, but some fraction will, and the result will be that an individual moves from S to I: remember that in SIR we assume that the disease passes on instantly. Let's refer to this as p_{infect}, the probability that an I will infect an S in a single contact. There are SI contacts in each timestep, of which a fraction p_{infect} will result in an infection. Putting this all together, the size of S will *reduce* by $p_{infect} SI$ (because the disease causes people to leave S by becoming infected).

If S is the number of susceptible people, we can denote the *change* in S by ΔS, the difference in S at each timestep. As the disease progresses we expect S to decrease: unless people enter the population from outside, the number of susceptible people only goes down since once someone has been infected they don't return to being susceptible again (having the disease makes you immune in this model). Mathematically we can say that

$$\Delta S = -p_{infect} SI$$

with the minus sign indicating that S is getting smaller.

The value p_{infect} is called a **parameter** of the model. The equations provide a description of the overall behaviour of the model. Within this, you can change the values of the parameters to explore the different kinds of behaviour possible within the model. You can make the disease more infectious by making p_{infect} larger, for example. It's often the case that, in models with several parameters (as SIR has), the values of the parameters will interact in interesting ways.

What about I? Every person who leaves S (and so ceases to be susceptible) becomes infected and so enters I. So we'd expect that the corresponding change in I, ΔI, would *increase* by the same amount as ΔS *decreased*, so as not to lose anyone from the population. But as well as contracting the disease, people also recover from it (or die): either way they are "removed" from the population affected by the disease.

(Whether you recover or die is obviously quite important to you, but in either event you are no longer infected or susceptible and so take no further part in the spread of the infection. Epidemic modelling can seem quite heartless at times.)

How many people are removed? SIR assumes that, just as a fraction p_{infect} of contacts result in infection, a fraction p_{remove} of infected individuals are removed. So the size of I is *increased* by susceptible people becoming infected, and *reduced* by infected people becoming removed. Putting this together we get

$$\Delta I = (p_{infect}\, SI) - (p_{remove}\, I)$$

The final step in the model is to account for removal, whereby the size of R increases at the same rate as that of I decreases.

$$\Delta R = p_{remove}\, I$$

And that's SIR: three equations that describe how the sizes of the three compartments change, and two parameters that define what fraction of contacts result in infections and what fraction of infections are removed in a given time period.

Looking at the maths, one can immediately deduce some things about how an SIR epidemic will progress. Firstly, as we mentioned, the size of S always decreases, while the size of R clearly always increases: the only place where anything

In the computational epidemiology and network science literatures the parameter we've called p_{infect} is usually denoted β, while p_{remove} is denoted α. It's easier to understand what's going on if we spell the meaning of the symbols out.

Compartmented models

interesting can happen is in the size of I, which both increases *and* decreases.

Secondly, the rate at which I increases depends on how big I is already: a larger value of I makes for a larger value of ΔI. But it's a bit more complicated than that, since it also depends on the size of S, where a smaller value of S means a smaller value of ΔI – and we know that S is always getting smaller. So these two terms – growing through infection and shrinking through removal – will fight it out as the disease progresses.

To summarise, we know that the sizes of S, I, and R will change over time. We know that S will shrink and R will grow, and I will... well, will do something that depends on the sizes of S and I. We also know that I grows at the same rate that S shrinks.

To find out exactly what happens, we need to explore these equations.

The computational model

To explore SIR, let's turn the mathematical model of three equations into a computational model that "runs the numbers" to show how the epidemic progresses.

We can represent each of the three changes in population directly as Python functions. Since they share the parameters p_{infect} and p_{remove}, we'll define them together using another function to which we pass the parameters and get back the change functions.

```python
def make_sir(pInfect, pRemove):
    # turn the equations into update functions
    def deltaS(S, I, R):
        return -pInfect * S * I
    def deltaI(S, I, R):
        return pInfect * S * I - pRemove * I
    def deltaR(S, I, R):
        return pRemove * I
```

(continues on next page)

(continued from previous page)

```
    # return the three functions
    return (deltaS, deltaI, deltaR)
```

We've used as far as possible the same names in the code as we
did in the maths: pInfect for p_{infect}, deltaS for ΔS, and so forth.
This will help keep things straight in our minds.

How do we "run" the epidemic? We've defined the ways in
which the sizes of the sub-populations change. If we start with
some initial sub-populations, we can then compute the change
and add it to the previous population to get the population at
the next timestep. We can do this repeatedly to trace out the
behaviour of the epidemic in time. The result will be a time
series for each sub-population tracking its size over time.

What should the initial sizes of the sub-populations be? Since
we're interested only in their sizes, we could say that given
N individuals a fraction $p_{infected}$ are initially infected, while
everyone else is susceptible: no-one starts off removed.

We can code this behaviour up as a single function.

This approach to
integration to get a time
series, known as the *direct*
or *Euler* method, isn't safe
in general, as it risks falling
foul of numerical instability
in the equations. There
are several more robust
solutions for the more
complex cases.

```
def epidemic_sir(T, N, pInfected, pInfect, pRemove):
    # create the change functions for these parameters
    (deltaS, deltaI, deltaR) = make_sir(pInfect, pRemove)

    # initial conditions
    sss = [ N * (1.0 - pInfected) ]
    iss = [ N * pInfected ]
    rss = [ 0 ]

    # push the initial conditions through the equations
    for t in range(1, T):
        # apply the change functions to the sub-populations of
        # the previous timestep to compute the changes
        ds = deltaS(sss[-1], iss[-1], rss[-1])
        di = deltaI(sss[-1], iss[-1], rss[-1])
        dr = deltaR(sss[-1], iss[-1], rss[-1])

        # the value at the next timestep are those at the
```

(continues on next page)

Compartmented models

(continued from previous page)

```
        # previous timestep plus the value of the change
        # in that value
        sss.append(sss[-1] + ds)
        iss.append(iss[-1] + di)
        rss.append(rss[-1] + dr)

    # return the time series
    return (list(range(0, T)), sss, iss, rss)
```

We need the initial conditions for the simulation: the population size (that won't change), the number of timesteps we want to run the simulation for, and the values of the three parameters pInfected, pInfect, and pRemove. For simplicity let's fix all these apart from pInfect. We'll start with 1/100th of the population infected (pInfected = 0.01), and 1/1000th of the infected population recovering in each timestep (pRemove = 0.001).

```
N = 1000
T = 5000
pInfected = 0.01
pRemove = 0.001
```

We can then choose different values of pInfect and see what the simulation shows us about the ways in which the sub-populations evolve.

```
import matplotlib
%matplotlib inline
%config InlineBackend.figure_format = 'png'
matplotlib.rcParams['figure.dpi'] = 300
import matplotlib.pyplot as plt
import seaborn
matplotlib.style.use('seaborn')
seaborn.set_context("notebook", font_scale=1.75)
```

```
epidemics = {}
for pInfect in [ 0.0000010, 0.0000020, 0.0000035,
                 0.0000040, 0.0000050, 0.0000080 ]:
    # run the epidemic equations
    epidemics[pInfect] = epidemic_sir(T, N, pInfected, pInfect,
→ pRemove)
```

(continues on next page)

The computational model

(continued from previous page)

```
(fig, axs) = plt.subplots(3, 2, sharex=True, sharey=True,
                          figsize=(12, 12))

# draw the sub-plots for selected values of pInfect
for (pInfect, ax) in [ (0.0000010, axs[0][0]),
                       (0.0000020, axs[0][1]),
                       (0.0000035, axs[1][0]),
                       (0.0000040, axs[1][1]),
                       (0.0000050, axs[2][0]),
                       (0.0000080, axs[2][1]) ]:
    (ts, sss, iss, rss) = epidemics[pInfect]

    # draw the graph in the sub-plot
    ax.plot(ts, sss, 'r-', label='suceptible')
    ax.plot(ts, iss, 'g-', label='infected')
    #ax.plot(ts, rss, 'k-', label='removed')
    ax.set_title('$p_{\\mathit{Infect}} = ' + '{b:.7f}$'.
→format(b=pInfect))
    ax.set_xlim([0, T])
    ax.set_ylim([0, N])

# fine-tune the figure
plt.suptitle('Progress of epidemic for different $p_{\\mathit
→{Infect}}$ ($p_{remove} = ' + '{a}$)'.format(a=pRemove))
for i in [0, 1, 2]:
    axs[i][0].set_ylabel('population that is...')
for i in[0, 1]:
    axs[1][i].set_xlabel('$t$')
axs[0][0].legend(loc='center left')
plt.show()
```

Compartmented models

Progress of epidemic for different p_{Infect} ($p_{remove} = 0.001$)

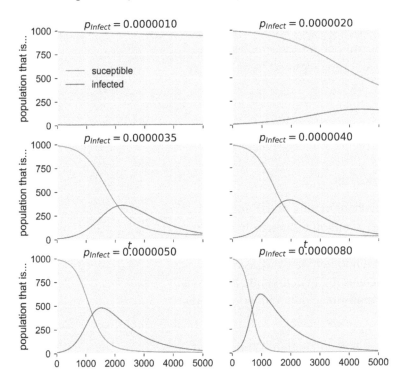

What are these graphs telling us? Start in the top left. At the start of the epidemic (when $t = 0$) we have a very small number of infected individuals and a very large number of susceptibles. The number of infecteds grows slowly as the time passes and the graph moves form left to right. But the disease is not very infectious: only 0.000001 of contacts leads to infection, just one in a million. At the start of the epidemic there are 990 susceptible people and 10 infected (1% of the total population), which means there can be at most 9900 susceptible-infected contacts. In the first timestep, then, the equations suggest that approximately 0.01 people become infected.

We can't infect two-hundredths of a person, of course: clearly it will take some time for there to be one new person infected. And once infections start people also start to recover, and the epidemic clearly never gets going.

We've engaged in some mathematical sleight-of-hand here, in that what we've described as a *discrete* model (of people being susceptible, infected, and so on) has then be treated as a *continuous* model that represents the sizes of compartments as real numbers. In order to work in this way the three SIR equations should really be be phrased as *differential* equations rather than as *difference* equations so that the passage from discrete to continuous time makes mathematical sense. The results obtained are the same in both cases, however.

But now look at the next diagrams. Even for very modest values of p_{infect} – 0.000002 to 0.000008 – we get considerable epidemics. At the peak of infections around 40–60% of the population is infected, compared to essentially no-one for the smallest value of p_{infect}. And that's with p_{infect} still tiny: eight contacts in every million resulting in an infection.

Consequences

Let those figures sink in for a moment.

The SIR model is telling us that changing the rate of infection from one in a million to eight in a million is enough to change the total proportion of infected people in a population from about 1% to about 60%! To put it another way, the process is very sensitive, and anything that changes the infection rate by even a miniscule amount can have an enormous, outsized, effect on the outbreak.

We have to be careful what we conclude, though. While we've got a "population" and some "contacts", we haven't said anything about the timescale over which we're talking: it's all been abstracted. So the "infection rate" is a somewhat notional concept that doesn't directly relate to *any* particular rate or disease in the real world. It's important to remember this and not draw any unsupported conclusions.

There *are* some conclusions that are supported, though. Firstly, we can see that the epidemic grows exponentially once it gets started. We can also see that it dies away exponentially after its peak. And we know that the population of infected people is a dynamic thing, with people recovering and new people being infected across the outbreak.

Compartmented models

Questions for discussion

- Look again at the graphs above. Are you surprised by them? Do they match how you think about, for example, winter flu?

- The numbers we've used in our model don't represent any particular disease. Do you think we could change that, so that our abstract model becomes more concrete? How might you do it?

Network models

One thing that may be bothering you about SIR is the idea
of a population where all the possible interactions between
individuals take place. You don't meet everyone in your city,
town, or village like that on a regular basis: that isn't how
societies work.

Admittedly you get this sort of "complete mixing" in *some*
scenarios. A school for young children (or, even better, a
toddler's nursery) perhaps works like this as the children go
out to play together and everyone mixes with everyone else. And
this is why diseases spread so rapidly through nurseries: one
sick child will infect all the others.

In chickenpox the infected
individual – almost always
a child – is latent for 7–10
days after exposure, but only
infectious for about 24 hours
before the symptoms (an
itchy rash) appear.

This phenomenon can be used constructively. When I was a
child it was commonplace for parents to hold "chickenpox
parties" and bring all the neighbouring children together to play
so they could be exposed – and then subsequently be immune
from further infection, since chickenpox confers very strong
immunity.

But in other cases the assumption of complete mixing is going
to break down. And since we know that even a small change
in infectivity can have a dramatic effect on the progress of an
epidemic, can we change SIR to accommodate the social realities
in which there are substantially fewer connections between
individuals that we might expect?

Networks

There are a couple of ways of answering this question, but the one we'll turn to here uses networks.

A **network** is simply a collection of **nodes** connected by **edges**. A road map is a good example of a network: the nodes are the road junctions, while the edges (which connect the junctions together) are the segments of roads. This is the reason we sometimes refer to the *road network*: it's a collection of (bits of) road that meet at various points.

The term **graph** is often used as a synonym for network.

Another good example of a network – and closer to our current application – is a **social network**. In a social network the nodes are people and the edges are "social links" or "social contacts" between them. While we usually think of social networks as being online, like Facebook or Twitter, the idea works in the real world too: when you meet your family, go shopping, go to work, or indulge in any of the activities of daily life you add edges to your social network between yourself and the people you meet. Typically the number of people you'll have social contact with will be considerably less than the entire population. The social network records the people with whom you have contact, and so in our application records people whom you might infect or be infected by.

Do the same thing for everyone in the population, and you have a social network for that population. The nodes are the individuals; the edges are the potentially infection-carrying social contacts. We can then simulate the progress of the epidemic over this network.

Complete networks

Suppose that, on your travels, you *did* actually happen to come into contact with everyone in the population, so that your social network had edges connecting you to everyone else. And suppose that everyone else did the same, so that everyone was connected to everyone. This is still a social network – a very dense one to be sure, perhaps like what happens on a nightclub dance floor. It also matches the assumptions we made earlier about complete mixing. So if we ran a simulation of disease spreading over this network, we'd presumably expect to see the same results as we did before.

Wouldn't we?

In the previous chapter we "pushed" an initial population of nodes through the equations. For a network we can do something slightly different. Each node represents an individual, so we have a colleciton of people whose evolution we can track through the SIR disease (rather than simply counting them). That will be useful later. But clearly there's more "book-keeping" to do in keeping track of everyone. It's harder, from a programming perspective, to model the disease on a network – but in doing so we gain a lot of flexibility, as we'll see later.

For the moment, we need to set up a computational simulation of the people and their connections. Fortunately there we have software than can help us do this.

```
import networkx
import epydemic
```

Since we're interested in the progress of an epidemic, we'll create an SIR process and then add some monitoring to get the same time series that we got for the continuous case.

```
class MonitoredSIR(epydemic.SIR, epydemic.Monitor):

    def __init__(self):
        super(MonitoredSIR, self).__init__()

    def build(self, params):
        '''Build the observation process.

        :param params: the experimental parameters'''
        super(MonitoredSIR, self).build(params)
```

(continues on next page)

(continued from previous page)

```
        # also monitor other compartments
        self.trackNodesInCompartment(epydemic.SIR.SUSCEPTIBLE)
        self.trackNodesInCompartment(epydemic.SIR.REMOVED)
```

We can now write a function to perform the simulation for
given parameters of pInfected, pInfect, and pRemove. For
completeness we'll also pass the function a network over which
to run the simulation. The function sets up the simulation using
epydemic, runs it, and extracts the results.

```
def network_sir(T, g, pInfected, pInfect, pRemove):
    # create the simulator
    m = MonitoredSIR()
    m.setMaximumTime(T)
    e = epydemic.SynchronousDynamics(m, g)

    # set the simulation parameters
    param = dict()
    param[epydemic.SIR.P_INFECTED] = pInfected
    param[epydemic.SIR.P_INFECT] = pInfect
    param[epydemic.SIR.P_REMOVE] = pRemove
    param[epydemic.Monitor.DELTA] = T / 50 # 50 samples

    # run the simulation
    rc = e.set(param).run()

    # extract the time series
    results = e.experimentalResults()[MonitoredSIR.TIMESERIES]
    ts = results[MonitoredSIR.OBSERVATIONS]
    sss = results[epydemic.SIR.SUSCEPTIBLE]
    iss = results[epydemic.SIR.INFECTED]
    rss = results[epydemic.SIR.REMOVED]

    # return the time series
    return(ts, sss, iss, rss)
```

To test our hypothesis, we need a complete "social network" to
operate over. Such networks are often called *complete graphs,* with
every node connected by an edge to every other.

```
g = networkx.complete_graph(N)
```

Finally we can run the equations *and* the network simulation and plot them together. If they generate the same results, we'd expect the two datasets to agree with each other.

```
fig = plt.figure(figsize=(8, 8))
ax = fig.gca()

pInfect = 0.000005      # chosen simply for illustration

# run the epidemic equations
(ts, sss, iss, rss) = epidemic_sir(T, N, pInfected, pInfect,
  ⌣pRemove)
ax.plot(ts, sss, 'r-', label='suceptible (theory)')
ax.plot(ts, iss, 'g-', label='infected (theory)')
#ax.plot(ts, rss, 'k-', label='removed (theory)')

# run the corresponding simulation
(sim_ts, sim_sss, sim_iss, sim_rss) = network_sir(T, g,
  ⌣pInfected, pInfect, pRemove)
ax.plot(sim_ts, sim_sss, 'rs', label='suceptible (simulation)')
ax.plot(sim_ts, sim_iss, 'gs', label='infected (simulation)')
#ax.plot(sim_ts, sim_rss, 'kx', label='removed (simulation)')

# fine-tune the figure
plt.title('Equations vs network ($p_{\\mathit{infect}} = ' + '
  ⌣{b:.7f}$, '.format(b=pInfect) + '$p_{remove} = ' + '{a}$)'.
  ⌣format(a=pRemove), y=1.05)
ax.set_xlabel('$t$')
ax.set_xlim([0, T])
ax.set_ylabel('population that is...')
ax.set_ylim([0, N])
ax.legend(loc='center right')
plt.savefig('network-same-beta-alpha.svg')
plt.show()
```

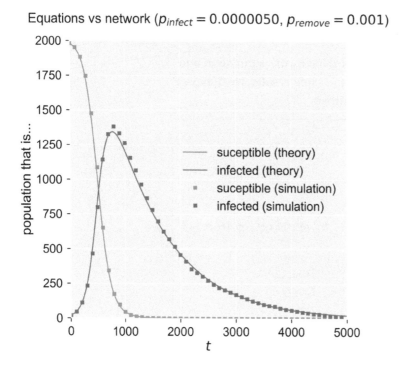

Equations vs network (p_{infect} = 0.0000050, p_{remove} = 0.001)

And so they do: the crosses of the simulation lie over the top of the solid lines of the SIR equations.

Not *exactly* over, for reasons we'll come to later.

The story so far

To recap, we defined SIR as a process and explored what happened in a scenario of complete mixing. We then reproduced these results in a different framework, with the same process running over a network, also with complete mixing. But clearly complete mixing isn't a good model of a social network: you don't meet everyone all the time, and therefore don't get exposed to all possible infected people.

Real social networks are very different: more "clumpy", more uneven, some people with more contacts than others. Everyone experiences this, and one would think that the differences (in the social contact structure) will make a difference to the epidemic (in the way it spreads). This is indeed the case, and we will

Network models

explore it later.

The simulation we ran above has two parts: the SIR process, and the network we ran it over – which in this case was a complete graph. We can of course change the network, and as we do we can explore how the disease behaves for different kinds of network. In the spirit of good science, we'll keep the disease the same, and only change the context in which it occurs, so that any changes we observe will be due to change in the network.

Questions for discussion

- We've now done two simulations of the same disease model: with equations, and with simulation. Which do you trust the results of more? Why?

- (For programmers.) How would you go about building a simulator for SIR?

Making fewer connections

If the complete graph is a representation of complete mixing, how do we represent "incomplete" mixing? With an *incomplete* graph, obviously...

Of course while there can only be one complete graph with a given number of nodes, once we start talking about incomplete graphs we have a huge number of options. We could have a network with *no* edges. (How would an epidemic spread over this network?) Or we could have a network that had a very uneven distribution of edges. Perhaps we could even extract a "real" social network from facebook or Twitter data.

The structure of a network is referred to mathematically as its **topology**. You can think of this as being "the way it's connected" What we're talking about, then, is exploring how the SIR process spreads over networks with different topologies.

Characterising a network's topology

Since we have a range of different topologies, we'll need some way of describing their properties so that we can tell them apart. There are a huge number of such **graph metrics** that have been developed, and we'll encounter a few of them in the course of this book. For the time being, we'll start with the most influential number, the **degree** of a node, which is simply the number of edges intersecting each node. Each node has its own degree. In your social network, the degree of the node that represents you

In the networks we'll be considering for now the degree of a node is fixed when the network is created. Later on when we encounter adaptive networks degree itself becomes a process that changes with time.

is simply the number of people you're connected to. The degree of a node is usually denoted k, for no particular reason.

$\langle k \rangle$ is usually pronounced "k mean".

For a given network we can enumerate the degrees of every node, but that's clearly not going to be very useful for a large network: you wouldn't be able to extract any useful information from the large list of numbers. But we can derive statistics from such lists. The most important is the **mean degree**, the "average" degree of a node, denoted $\langle k \rangle$. While the degree of every node has to be an integer (you can't have half a friend), the mean degree of the population overall will typically be a real number.

For the complete graph every node has exactly the same degree, being one less that the number of nodes in the network, since there's an edge between every node and every other (except itself). This means that k is always $(N-1)$ for every node, and therefore so is $\langle k \rangle$.

In general things will be more complicated. The degrees of nodes in a network form a **degree distribution**, which we can plot as a histogram to show the number of nodes with each degree (we do this below). If we use N to represent the number of nodes in the network, we'll use N_k to represent the number of nodes with degree k. Then we can compute $\langle k \rangle$ very easily from this distibution, by summing up the numbers of ndoes with each degree and then dividing by the number of nodes.

If this use of the word "distribution" sounds like it should be connected to probability theory – it is. The degree histogram shows the relative numbers of nodes with each different degree, and so defines the probability of randomly choosing a node with degree k. $\langle k \rangle$ is then the expected value of the degree.

$$\langle k \rangle = \frac{\sum_k N_k}{N}$$

There are a lot of other metrics that we could consider, but the degree distribution is the most important and well-studied. It's not the whole story, however, because there are will be a *lot* of different networks with the *same* degree distribution and mean degree, depending on exactly how the edges that intersect each node connect to other nodes. So while one side of network toppology is captured by statistics, there's another side that concerns the details of which nodes are **adjacent** to each other by having an edge between them: it matters *who* your friends are, not just **how many** you have. We sometimes call the set of nodes adjacent to a node its **neighbours**.

Making fewer connections

ER networks

Let's start with one of the simplest non-complete topologies. This topology was initially explored in depth in the late 1950's by Paul Erdős and Alfred Rényi [9]. They called their approach "random graphs", but that's a slightly misleading name: we can produce "random" networks with *any* topology as we saw above. Fortunately the influence of Erdős and Rényi has been so profound that networks of this type are now referred to as **Erdős-Rényi** or **ER networks**.

[9] Paul Erdős and Alfred Renyi. On random graphs. *Publicationes Mathematicæ*, 6:290–297, 1959

(Paul Erdős (pronounced "AIR-dish") was the most prolific mathematician of the 20th century. A peripatetic genius, he owned essentially nothing and travelled between university mathematics schools seeking problems to work on. He's also very "central" in the network of mathematical co-authors, where someone's "Erdős number" measures the number of co-authorships between them and Erdős. (Smaller in better.) His biography [10] provides a fascinating insight into mathematical life.)

Alfred Rényi, the other half of the partnership, was a noted mathematician whose very significant other work has been rather overshadowed by his wonderfully productive association with Erdős. He was responsible for the definition of a mathematician as "a machine for turning coffee into theorems".

[10] Paul Hoffman. *The man who loved only numbers: The story of Paul Erdőos and the search for mathematical truth.* Hyperion, 1998

The idea of an ER network is that there exists an edge between any pair of nodes with some fixed probability, and the existence of any edge is independent of the existence of any other.

Building ER networks

Again, in the literature p_{edge} is usually denoted ϕ.

From this simple description of the degree distribution, an ER network is also very simple to build. Pick a number of nodes N, and build the complete graph K_N. Remember that the complete graph has an edge between every pair of nodes. Now pick a parameter p_{edge} between 0 and 1. Work through all the edges, and for each edge pick a random number s between 0 and 1. If $s \leq p_{edge}$ then keep the edge; if $s > p_{edge}$, remove it. You'll end up with a network in which there's an edge between each pair of nodes with a probability p_{edge}. If $p_{edge} = 1$ we have the complete graph (we *always* keep an edge); if $p_{edge} = 0$ we have the empty graph (we *never* keep an edge); and for values in between we have a more or less sparse collection of edges.

Drawing the result can help get the idea straight.

```python
(fig, axs) = plt.subplots(3, 2, sharex=True, sharey=True,
                          figsize=(12, 18))

# a small network to visualise
N = 20

# draw the network for different values of phi
for (phi, ax) in [ (0.05, axs[0][0]),
                   (0.10, axs[0][1]),
                   (0.25, axs[1][0]),
                   (0.50, axs[1][1]),
                   (0.75, axs[2][0]),
                   (0.99, axs[2][1]) ]:
    # create a random ER network
    G = networkx.erdos_renyi_graph(N, phi)

    # draw the network in the sub-plot
    networkx.draw_circular(G, ax=ax)
    ax.set_title('$p_{edge} = ' + '{p}$'.format(p=phi))

# fine-tune the figure
plt.suptitle('ER networks for different values of $p_{edge}$ '
 + '($N = {n}$)'.format(n=N))
plt.show()
```

ER networks for different values of p_{edge} ($N = 20$)

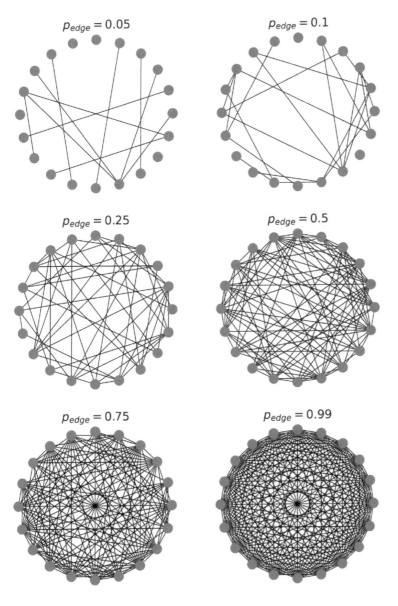

At the top left where p_{edge} is small, we have very few edges: 5% of the possible total, in fact. As we progress towards the bottom right the network gets more and more dense, until at 99% of

We sometimes denote the ER network with N nodes and a connection probability p_{edge} by $G_{N,p_{edge}}$.

the possible edges it's quite hard to spot that any are actually missing at all.

What is $\langle k \rangle$ for this topology? The answer turns out to be quite simple. An ER network has $\langle k \rangle = \frac{p_{edge}}{N}$. Moreover the degree distribution – the number of nodes with more, or less, edges than the mean, is a **normal** distribution, the "bell curve" we see in many phenomena.

```python
fig = plt.figure(figsize=(8, 8))
ax = fig.gca()

# a sample network
N = 10000
kmean = 40
phi = (kmean + 0.0) / N

# build the network
g = networkx.gnp_random_graph(N, phi)
#G = networkx.erdos_renyi_graph(N, phi)

# draw the degree distribution
ks = list(dict(networkx.degree(g)).values())
ax.hist(ks, bins=max(ks))
ax.set_title('ER network degree distribution ($N = {n}, \\
 ↪langle k \\rangle = {k}'.format(n=N, k=kmean) + ', p_{edge}
 ↪= ' + '{p}$)'.format(p=phi), y=1.05)
ax.set_xlabel('$k$')
ax.set_ylabel('$N_k$')

plt.savefig('degree-distribution-er.png')
plt.show()
```

ER network degree distribution ($N = 10000$, $\langle k \rangle = 40$, $p_{edge} = 0.004$)

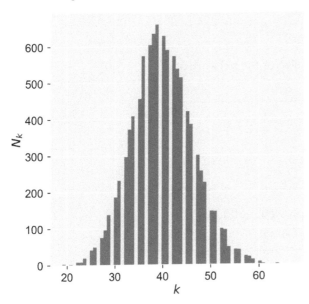

So about one-third of the nodes (about 675) have a degree around the mean (40), with the number of nodes having more (or less) neighbours dropping off on either side of the mean. There are very few nodes with degrees in single figures, and very few with degrees of twice the mean – and none with really large degree. In fact for any network there will be a **minimum degree** k_{min} and a **maximum degree** k_{max}. The ER network's degree distribution says that the maximum degree is never "too far" from the mean.

Epidemic spreading on ER networks

After all that network science we can finally ask ourselves a disease-related question: what happens as we vary $\langle k \rangle$? We already know that when $\langle k \rangle = (N-1)$ the network has complete mixing. But what happens as $\langle k \rangle$ gets *smaller* – that is, people have fewer and fewer contacts with each other – for the *same* disease? We'd presumably expect that fewer people will become infected overall, which also suggests that at some point the

From now on we'll mainly use $\langle k \rangle$ as the parameter for ER networks rather than ϕ: we can convert between them easily, and $\langle k \rangle$ is a more intuitive idea.

disease will simply die out without affecting very many people at all.

Let's see.

We'll take the same parameters for the size of the network and the disease that we had before.

```
N = 2000
T = 5000
pInfected = 0.01
pInfect = 0.0001
pRemove = 0.001
```

But instead of building a complete graph we'll build ER networks and see what happens as we change $\langle k \rangle$.

```
epidemics = {}
for kmean in [ 10, 20, 30, 40, 50, 100 ]:
    # create an ER network
    phi = (kmean + 0.0) / N
    g = networkx.gnp_random_graph(N, phi)

    # run the corresponding simulation
    epidemics[kmean] = network_sir(T, g, pInfected, pInfect,
    ⌐pRemove)
```

```
(fig, axs) = plt.subplots(3, 2, sharex=True, sharey=True,
⌐figsize=(12, 15))

# draw sub-plots for the different values of kmean
for (kmean, ax) in [ (10,  axs[0][0]),
                     (20,  axs[0][1]),
                     (30,  axs[1][0]),
                     (40,  axs[1][1]),
                     (50,  axs[2][0]),
                     (100, axs[2][1]) ]:
    (sim_ts, sim_sss, sim_iss, sim_rss) = epidemics[kmean]
    ax.plot(sim_ts, sim_sss, 'r.', label='suceptible')
    ax.plot(sim_ts, sim_iss, 'g.', label='infected')
    ax.set_title('$\\langle k \\rangle = {k}$'.format(k=kmean))
    ax.set_xlim([0, T])
    ax.set_ylim([0, N])
```

(continues on next page)

Making fewer connections

(continued from previous page)

```
# fine-tune the figure
plt.suptitle('SIR over ER networks ($N = {n}'.format(n=N) + ',␣
  →p_{\\mathit{Infect}} = ' + '{b:.4f}'.format(b=pInfect) + ',␣
  →p_{remove} = ' + '{a}$)'.format(a=pRemove))
for i in [0, 1, 2]:
    axs[i][0].set_ylabel('population that is...')
for i in[0, 1]:
    axs[2][i].set_xlabel('$t$')
axs[0][0].legend(loc='center right')
plt.show()
```

SIR over ER networks ($N = 2000, p_{Infect} = 0.0001, p_{remove} = 0.001$)

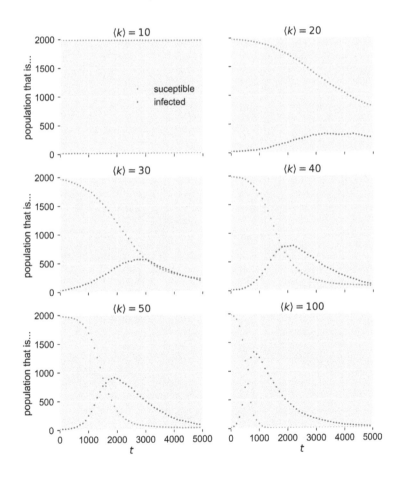

Compare these graphs to the ones earlier and you'll see the same shapes: changing $\langle k \rangle$ has the same effect as changing p_{infect} in terms of moving the peak of infections.

Questions for discussion

- In a network model two people are either connected, or they aren't. Is that realistic? Could we change our model to make it reflect different "strengths of connection"? What might that let us do?

- We say above that "changing $\langle k \rangle$ has the same effect as changing p_{infect}". Can you put that in less mathematical terms? What does it mean?

Contact tracing

Let's now turn to a more detailed look at how an epidemic spreads, and in particular to the subject of who infects whom. Working this out is the subject of **contact tracing**, which is the process of determining the infection history as the disease passes through the population. In an SIR infection this boils down to deducing the pattern of infected individuals over the course of the disease.

The point of contact tracing is three-fold:

1. It provides **data**: how many people have been infected in the population? how many were not infected even though they were in contact with an infected individual? and so forth.

2. It allows **treatment** of the infected individuals, possibly before they are symptomatic.

3. It allows **countermeasures** to be deployed to reduce the spread of the diseaase.

In a real epidemic the data-collection aspect is vital, since we will often now know how contagious a new disease is. The treatment aspect is also vitally important for the individuals concerned, since early treatment is often more effective. And for many diseases there will be effective countermeasures such as quarantine that can be imposed to reduce the disease's spread even further. (We should really consider treatment to be a countermeasure at the population level, since treated individuals will probably spread the disease less than the untreated.)

However, contact tracing in a real epidemic is a laborious process. We need to identify infected people, either by testing them or by observation of their symptoms, if these are sufficiently distinct to permit definitive identification. Then we need to identify all those with whom they have been in contact (their contact network) and test (or observe) *them* to determine if they are infected – and then repeat the process with *their* contact network, and so forth.

Fortunately, in a simulated epidemic, all the information we need is directly available. We know the contact network *a priori*, and can instrument our simulation to determine the ways in which individuals were infected. We can then use this instrumented model as a basis for studying disease dynamics, treatment strategies, and other countermeasures.

Progress of an epidemic

Most diseases that spread by contact share a remarkable property: if you have the disease, *someone gave it to you*: exactly one person. Contrary to the notion in earlier ages that all diseases resulted from "bad air", in many cases pathogens pass from one person to another by fairly direct contact. Each contact offers the possibility of infection from one person to another.

In the case of malaria the name itself reflects this idea, being derived from the Italian *mala aria*, "bad air".

This is a simplification, of course. Some disease are airborne, or leave long-lived traces on furniture or objects from which they can be picked up. If a lot of infected people move through the same space, they increase the "load" of pathogens in the space and so make infection more likely – and also mask who it was who actually did the infecting. But for the sorts of infections we're currently considering we assume that they pass person to person.

What, then, does the spread of the disease through the population look like?

Let's simplify a little more and assume we have a single infected person within a wholly susceptible population. How does the infection spread? Let's trace the infection as it progresses. We'll do this a little more "manually" than we have done previously, just to make the mechanism more explicit.

Compare this to the description of SIR earlier.

We first create a small ER network and "seed" it with a single infected person, which we store in the network itself as an attribute. We then step through time and at each step look at the neighbours of each infected node. If they are susceptible, we infect them with some probability and – if they become infected – we record their infection for the next timestap. We also mark the edge that the infection traversed.

```python
def stepEpidemic(g):
    # keep track of progress in this timestep
    inf = []

    # extract all the infected ndoes
    infecteds = [ n for n in g.nodes
                    if 'infected' in g.nodes[n].keys() ]

    # advance the epidemic
    for n in infecteds:
        infs = []
        if 'infected' in g.nodes[n].keys():
            # infect every susceptible neighbour
            # with probability pInfect
            for m in g.neighbors(n):
                # ignore already-infected neighbours
                if 'infected' not in g.nodes[m].keys():
                    # decide whether to infect or not
                    if numpy.random.random() < pInfect:
                        # we're infecting, record this
                        # and the edge the infection traversed
                        g.nodes[m]['infected'] = True
                        infs.append(m)
                        g.edges[n, m]['occupied'] = True

        # record the infection mapping
        if len(infs) > 0:
            inf.append((n, infs))

    # return the mapping of who infected whom
    return inf
```

We can then draw the progress of the infection over the network
as time progresses.

```python
def drawEpidemic(g, ax, t):
    # compute node colours
    inf = 0
    nodes = list(g.nodes)
    ncs = [ 'blue' ] * len(nodes)
    for i in range(len(nodes)):
        n = nodes[i]
        if 'infected' in g.nodes[n].keys():
            ncs[i] = 'red'
            inf += 1

    # compute edge colours
    edges = list(g.edges)
    ecs = [ 'black' ] * len(edges)
    for i in range(len(edges)):
        (n, m) = edges[i]
        if 'occupied' in g.edges[n, m].keys():
            ecs[i] = 'red'

    # draw the contact tree
    networkx.draw_circular(g, ax=ax,
                           node_color=ncs, edge_color=ecs)
    ax.set_title('$t = {t}, [I] = {i}$'.format(t=t, i=inf))

(fig, axs) = plt.subplots(3, 2, figsize=(12, 18))

# build a small ER contact network
N = 20
pEdge = 0.25
g = networkx.gnp_random_graph(N, pEdge)

# infect a single person
g.nodes[0]['infected'] = True
infs = [ [ (None, [ 0 ]) ] ]

pInfect = 0.19

t = 0
for x in range(3):
    for y in range(2):
```

(continues on next page)

(continued from previous page)

```
        # draw the infected nodes and tramission edges
        ax = axs[x][y]
        drawEpidemic(g, ax, t)

        # advance the epidemic
        infs.append(stepEpidemic(g))
        t += 1

# fine-tune the figure
plt.suptitle('Progress of an epidemic ($p_{\\mathit{infect}} =
↪' + '{i})$'.format(i=pInfect))
plt.show()
```

Progress of an epidemic ($p_{infect} = 0.19$)

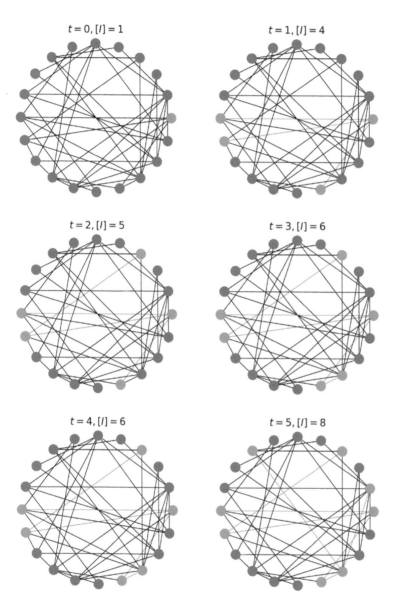

$t = 0, [I] = 1$

$t = 1, [I] = 4$

$t = 2, [I] = 5$

$t = 3, [I] = 6$

$t = 4, [I] = 6$

$t = 5, [I] = 8$

There are several things to note here. Firstly, look how fast the number of infected (denoted $[I]$ in the figures) people increases! The disease rapidly goes from being somewhere to being *everywhere,* and just explodes as grows: the rate at which it spreads increases as the proportion of infected people increases, which is the essential characteristic of exponential growth.

Secondly, notice how few edges were traversed. This makes sense, because there can only be one "transmission" edge for every node, which will only be a small fraction of the total nodes.

Contact trees

We can make this clearer by drawing the process slightly differently. Instead of drawing the network as a whole and showing the way the infection spreads, we'll focus on the infected nodes only and show how they relate – in other words, who affected whom.

We start at $t = 0$ with one infected node. At the next timestep we'll draw a second line of nodes that were infected by this node, connected to it by edges. In the next timestep we'll draw a third line of those who were infected by *those* nodes, and so on as time progresses.

```python
def drawContactTree(ax, t, ct):
    # turn the infection list into a network
    g = networkx.Graph()
    for infs in ct:
        for (n, ms) in infs:
            for m in ms:
                g.add_node(m)
                if n is not None:
                    g.add_edge(n, m)

    # compute the layers in the tree and the number of
    # infections from each individual
    secondaries = dict()
    ns = [ 0 ]
    layers = [ ns ]
    while len(ns) > 0:
        layer = []
```

(continues on next page)

Contact trees

(continued from previous page)

```python
        for n in ns:
            gs = set(g.neighbors(n))
            if len(layers) > 1:
                gs -= set(layers[-2])
            layer.append(list(gs))
            if len(gs) > 0:
                secondaries[n] = len(gs)
        ns = [n for cs in layer for n in cs]
        if len(ns) > 0:
            layers.append(ns)

    # compute locations
    pos = dict()
    dy = 1.0 / (len(layers) + 1)
    y = 1.0 - dy / 2
    for layer in layers:
        dx = 1.0 / (len(layer) + 1)
        x = dx
        for n in layer:
            pos[n] = (x, y)
            x += dx
        y -= dy

    # compute R_t
    if len(secondaries.keys()) > 0:
        Rt = sum(secondaries.values()) / len(secondaries.
↪keys())
    else:
        Rt = 0

    # draw the tree
    networkx.draw_networkx(g, pos, ax=ax,
                           node_color='red', with_labels=False)
    ax.set_xlim([0, 1])
    ax.set_ylim([0, 1])
    ax.axis('off')
    ax.set_title('$t = {t}, R = {rt:.2f}$'.format(t=t, rt=Rt))

(fig, axs) = plt.subplots(3, 2, figsize=(12, 12))

t = 0
for x in range(3):
```

(continues on next page)

(continued from previous page)

```
    for y in range(2):
        ax = axs[x][y]
        layers = infs[:(t + 1)]
        drawContactTree(ax, t, layers)
        t += 1

# fine-tune the figure
plt.suptitle('Progress of an epidemic ($p_{\\mathit{infect}} =
 ' + '{i})$'.format(i=pInfect))
plt.show()
```

Progress of an epidemic ($p_{infect} = 0.19$)

$t = 0, R = 0.00$ $t = 1, R = 3.00$

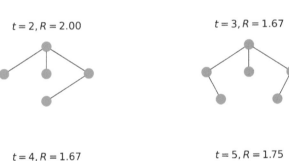

$t = 2, R = 2.00$ $t = 3, R = 1.67$

$t = 4, R = 1.67$ $t = 5, R = 1.75$

This layered structure is a **contact tree**. The topmost node is
patient zero, the first person infected in the epidemic. Those
in the next layer down are the first set of secondary cases, the

individuals infected by patient zero. And so on. Notice that because a node stays infected (in this very simple model) it may continue to infect nodes, so the layers can grow over time as more secondary cases occur from each infected.

You'll notice that in the above diagram R goes *down* over time. Why is that? It's because each individual can only be infected once and, once infected, can't be infected again. Later infected individuals are therefore increasingly likely to have neighbours who are already infected, and so have less opportunity to pass on the disease to new people. This phenomenon of the network "filling up" with infected individuals – and later, in SIR, with those who've been removed – is why epidemics die out naturally without necessarily infecting the entire population. It's also the basis for vaccination, which is a topic we'll return to later.

Computer scientists refer to the top-most node of a tree as the **root**, and always draw the root at the *top* of a tree diagram. Don't ask me why.

Questions for discussion

- Suppose you're been put in charge of tracking and tracing people's contacts. How would you do it? Is there any technology that would make the job easier?

- Tracing contacts is quite invasive of people's privacy. Is it justified when there's an epidemic happening? How about in "normal" circumstances?

Epidemic threshold

We're familiar with the idea that some diseases are more infectious than others. In real-world epidemics this is embodied in the case reproduction number $\mathcal{R}$, which counts the number of secondary infections arising on average from every primary infection. In network-based modelling it is embodied in p_{infect}, the probability that a contact leads to an infection.

But how infectious does a disease have to be to cause an epidemic? – that is to say, to create infection in a sizeable fraction of a population?

Clearly these two ideas are related: a disease that passes easily between people will be more likely to pass to more people. But it turns out that the relationship isn't as simple as we might expect. It's affected by a number of factors, including the disease parameters and the topology of the network – in other words, by the disease *and* the environment in which it finds itself. This is important: we're limited in what we can do about the basic infectiousness of a disease since that's defined by its biology, but the significance of topology opens-up the possibilty of countermeasures at a population level.

Looking back at the SIR model on an ER network, we see patterns in the way it spreads. For very low values of $\langle k \rangle$, the mean degree of the network, the epidemic never really "gets going". We can think of this as being what happens when the disease begins in population that's too disconnected to spread the disease before the infected individuals recover (or die).

We don't see this phenoemnon in continuous (non-network) compartmented models, in which *every* infection results in an epidemic of some size. This shows that the network approach is capturing something interesting: it lets is see phenomena that are absent from other models.

This is the other extreme to the fully connected network where *all* connections are in play and the propagation of the disease depends solely on the relationship between the rates of infection and recovery.

Let's ask a different question, though. If we fix the topology but change the infectivity, what happens to the numbers of people infected? We already know that in the fully-mixed case a very small change in infectivity results in a massive change in the size of the epidemic. But that was in a somewhat unrealistic case.

A related question is: for a particular topology, is there a characteristic degree of infectiousness that's needed to start an epidemic, below which one doesn't occur? To put it another way, is there an **epidemic threshold** that a disease on a network must exceed before it can go epidemic?

The epidemic threshold of an ER network

Let's look at the case for an ER network, the simplest model we have. (We've already accepted that it's not a great model of human contact networks, but we'll refine this later.)

To locate the epidemic threshold (assuming it exists), we need to simulate epidemics on networks across a range of infectiousness – that is to say, for different values of p_{infect}. If we want to test, shall we say, 50 different values of p_{infect} we'll need to run at least 50 experiments, one per value.

But we know there's a lot of randomness going on as well. The networks we create are random; we seed them randomly with infected individuals; and the disease progression is itself a random or stochastic process. What if, by chance, we chose as the seed individuals a group of people who were all right next to each other, with few other people to infect? Alternatively, what if, by chance, the infection failed to transmit a large number of times, and so died out?

There are a number of ways to deal with these issues, but the safest, most general, and most straightforward one is to conduct lots of trials and look at the patterns in the results, possibly then taking averages of the trials to find the "expected result" for a given value of p_{infect}. By repeating the experiment we reduce the influence of chances that "unlikely" combinations of circumstances will sway the answer. A suitably large number of repetitions will often allow us to squeeze out the variance in the results of the individual simulations.

The disadvantage of this approach is that it involves doing a lot more simulation, which in turn requires more computing power. Fortunately the scale of compute power we need is readily available nowadays, and we can conduct experiments using "clusters" of computers configured identically and each performing a share of the experiments we need doing.

To professional researchers, anyway: not so much for hobby use, although cloud computing provides access to fairly affordable computing resources.

```
lab = epyc.ClusterLab(profile='hogun',
                    notebook=epyc.JSONLabNotebook('datasets/
 ⌐threshold-er.json'))
with lab.sync_imports():
    import time
    import networkx
    import epyc
    import epydemic
    import numpy
print('{n} engines available'.format(n = lab.
 ⌐numberOfEngines()))
```

```
importing time on engine(s)
importing networkx on engine(s)
importing epyc on engine(s)
importing epydemic on engine(s)
importing numpy on engine(s)
importing mpmath on engine(s)
72 engines available
```

```
# from https://nbviewer.jupyter.org/gist/minrk/4470122
def pxlocal(line, cell):
    ip = get_ipython()
    ip.run_cell_magic("px", line, cell)
    ip.run_cell(cell)
```

(continues on next page)

The epidemic threshold of an ER network

(continued from previous page)

```
get_ipython().register_magic_function(pxlocal, "cell")
```

Because we're wanting to create a lot of random networks, we'll add code to the computational experiment to create them as required. Otherwise we'd run the risk of doing too many experiments on the same random network, and being affected by any features it happened to have.

```
%%pxlocal

class ERNetworkDynamics(epydemic.StochasticDynamics):

    # Experimental parameters
    N = 'N'
    KMEAN = 'kmean'

    def __init__(self, p):
        super(ERNetworkDynamics, self).__init__(p)

    def configure(self, params):
        super(ERNetworkDynamics, self).configure(params)

        # build a random ER network with the given parameters
        N = params[self.N]
        kmean = params[self.KMEAN]
        pEdge = (kmean + 0.09) / N
        g = networkx.gnp_random_graph(N, pEdge)
        self.setNetworkPrototype(g)
```

We will conduct our exploration on the same sort of network we've used before – 10^4 nodes with $\langle k \rangle = 40$ – over 50 values of p_{infect}.

```
# test network
lab[ERNetworkDynamics.N] = 10000
lab[ERNetworkDynamics.KMEAN] = 40

# disease parameters
lab[epydemic.SIR.P_INFECTED] = 0.001
lab[epydemic.SIR.P_REMOVE] = 0.002
```

(continues on next page)

(continued from previous page)

```
lab[epydemic.SIR.P_INFECT] = numpy.linspace(0.00001, 0.0002,
                                            num=50)
```

Finally, we'll set up the number of repetitions. For each point
in the space we'll create 10 random networks and run the
experiment 10 times on each, re-seeding the network randomly
with infected individuals each time.

```
m = epydemic.SIR()
e = ERNetworkDynamics(m)
rc = lab.runExperiment(epyc.RepeatedExperiment(
                       epyc.RepeatedExperiment(e, 10),
                       10))
```

A lot of computation now ensues, and eventually we get the
results back.

```
df = epyc.JSONLabNotebook('datasets/threshold-er.json').
 ⌐dataframe()
```

We can now look at the data. Let's begin by plotting the results
of *all* the experiments we did – 5000 datapoints in all – to see
that shape of the results.

```
fig = plt.figure(figsize=(8, 8))
ax = fig.gca()

# plot the size of the removed population
ax.plot(df[epydemic.SIR.P_INFECT],
        df[epydemic.SIR.REMOVED], 'r.')
ax.set_xlabel('$p_{\\mathit{infect}}$')
ax.set_ylabel('population that is...')
ax.set_title('Epidemic size vs $p_{\\mathit{infect}}$', y=1.05)

plt.show()
```

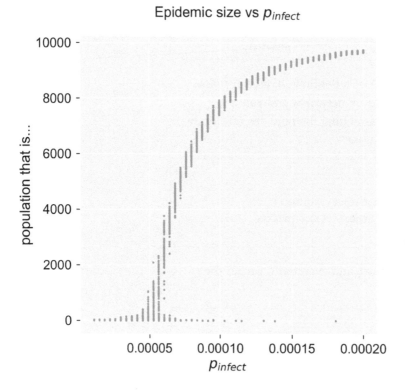

What does this show? Unlike many graphs we see, there are several points corresponding to each value of p_{infect}, each representing the result of a single simulation. The height of the "line" formed by these points is larger for those parameter values that show the highest variance.

At the two extremes of the curve it's easy to interpret what's going on. Low infectivity (at the left) means that almost none of the poopulation becomes infected, as the disease dies out quickly. High infectivity (at the right) causes almost all the population to become infected – although not quite all, it would seem.

But what about the middle part of the curve, between these extrema? There are two things to notice. Firstly, for each value of p_{infect}, there's substantially more variance. This is the essence of a stochastic process: you can get different results for the same starting conditions. Remember, we did 10 experiments on each random network and still get different answers, so there's something inherently variable at work. But secondly, notice that for most of the values of p_{infect} the results are "clustered" into a small line. Remember that we ran experiments on 10 different networks, so there's clearly also some commonality at work in the process where it gives closely-related (but different) results for different networks and seeds of infection, even though there's still variance.

Let's zoom-in on part of the curve so see the variation in more detail.

```python
fig = plt.figure(figsize=(8, 8))
ax = fig.gca()

# plot the size of the removed population
pInfects = df[[pInfect > 0.00003 and pInfect < 0.00008
                for pInfect in df[epydemic.SIR.P_INFECT]]]
ax.plot(pInfects[epydemic.SIR.P_INFECT],
        pInfects[epydemic.SIR.REMOVED], 'r.')
ax.set_xlabel('$p_{\\mathit{infect}}$')
ax.set_ylabel('population that is...')
ax.set_title('Epidemic size vs $p_{\\mathit{infect}}$ (detail)
 ↵', y=1.05)

plt.show()
```

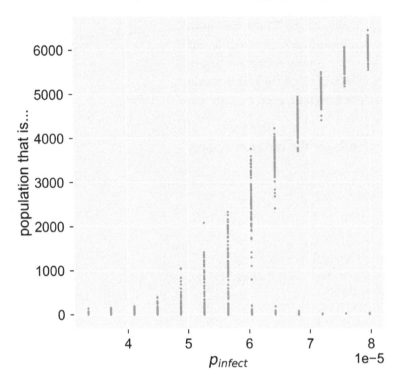

Epidemic size vs p_{infect} (detail)

As p_{infect} increases the possible sizes of the epidemic start to vary, from nothing up to maybe a thousand people. As we keep increasing p_{infect} the range keeps increasing, but still with some instances of the epidemic not getting started. This is shown by the columns of points becoming rather "stretched-out": sometimes we get an epidemic of about 4000, sometimes we get zero. As we *keep* increasing p_{infect} the epidemic starts being consistently larger, with a smaller chance of it failing to take hold, and the size starts to become more consistent as well: the variance goes down. Eventually we have a situation in which around 98% of the experiments result in an epidemic that infects around 60% of the population.

We can look at this data slightly differently, by plotting the average size of the epidemic for each value of p_{infect}: the average of our 100 experiments. But we should also keep track of the

Error bars usually show the standard deviation (also called the standard error) of the dataset at that point.

errors, and the standard way of doing this is to include error bars on the plot.

```python
fig = plt.figure(figsize=(8, 8))
ax = fig.gca()

# plot the size of the removed population
pInfects = sorted(df[epydemic.SIR.P_INFECT].unique())
repetitions = int(len(df[epydemic.SIR.P_INFECT]) /
 ↪len(pInfects))
removeds = []
stdErrors = []
for pInfect in pInfects:
    removeds.append(df[df[epydemic.SIR.P_INFECT] ==
 ↪pInfect][epydemic.SIR.REMOVED].mean())
    stdErrors.append(df[df[epydemic.SIR.P_INFECT] ==
 ↪pInfect][epydemic.SIR.REMOVED].std())
ax.errorbar(pInfects, removeds, yerr=stdErrors, fmt='r-',
 ↪ecolor='0.75', capsize=2.0)
ax.set_xlabel('$p_{\\mathit{infect}}$')
ax.set_ylabel('population that is...')
ax.set_title('Epidemic size vs $p_{\\mathit{infect}}$' + ',
 ↪mean of {r} repetitions'.format(r=repetitions), y=1.05)

plt.show()
```

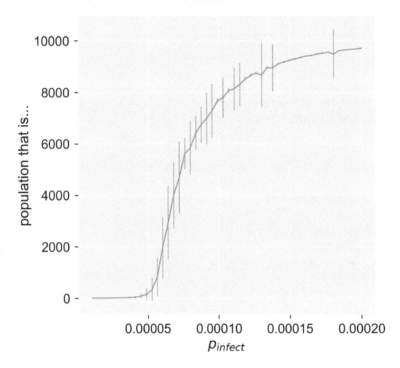

Epidemic size vs p_{infect}, mean of 100 repetitions

So there's still a lot of variance in the results. The error bars just present the same information in a terms of summary statistics like mean and variance. We can also see that the variance changes quite considerably: there's variance in the variance. Both of these suggest that we should do more experiments to see whether the values converge more closely to cluster around their mean. One advantage of simulation is that we can easily do exactly this, simply by crunching more numbers – a luxury not present in real-world epidemiology.

The "variance of the variance" is also called the *skewness*.

But even if the results do cluster more tightly around the mean, we know from plotting the "raw" results that there's an important pattern at work by which sometimes, even for infectious disieases, an epidemic fails to happen. This information has been *completely lost* in the plot of summary statistics: there's nothing to suggest that a zero-sized epidemic is a possible result. There are ways to present summary statistics that do show this, but it's important to realise that averaging by its natire hides detail – and that detail may be important.

Questions for discussion

- Where is all this variance coming from? – aren't we getting exact answers by running simulations in a computer?

- The existence of an epidemic threshold suggests that some diseases never become epidemics. Is that right?

Human contact networks

Since we now know that the structure of a network can affect the way a disease behaves, the obvious question is exactly what this effect is. A related question, somewhat less abstract, is how this effect manifests itself on a more realistic model of human contacts. If we can develop a model that mimics a "real" social situation, we can get closer to how real epidemics may behave.

Unsurprisingly, modelling human contacts is quite hard. Indeed, there is as yet no scientific consensus on what sorts of networks are the "best" model – not least because there are lots of different social structures to account for. A city is not just a large village: the ways in which people mix change fundamentally as the geographic and population scales increase, when you no longer know your neighbours and when you travel and mix over a wider area. Even such a simple sentence implies a lot of mathematical complexity. There is less mixing on a small scale with neighbours, but more mixing at longer distances with non-neighbours – and this is before we consider how friendship networks interrelate, and the effects of disease countermeasures such as social distancing that suddenly became a feature of modern life.

Suffice it to say that the study of contact networks is still an active field of research, being conducted experimentally by the study of real-world social networks as exposed by social media, and theoretically by the study of networks with topological structures that try to reflect how people interact.

While the "right" model is not yet known, we can still make progress by making use of (what we claim is) a better model than the simple ER network, and explore what effects it has.

Social structures

A human contact network has to model the structures we actually find in human social structures. These structures have been studied extensively [11,12], and they exhibit huge variation – far more than we find in, for example, the structure of networks in natural physical and biological systems. This is perhaps due to the diversity of cultural factors that drive social structures, or perhaps because a lot of such networks have been designed for specific purposes rather than simply evolving at random.

One common factor is that the degree distribution of a contact network is not normal (in the mathematical sense) like that of an ER network. Instead of the number of contacts clustering around a mean, we tend to observe a small number of nodes who are very highly connected – far more connected than is possible in an ER network. These people are sometimes referred to as "hubs" [13]. In disease modelling, "super-spreaders" might be a better term: individuals who, if they become infected, can potentially infect a huge number of others. This has implications for countermeasures and for vaccination, as we'll see later.

Contact networks often also exaggerate factors that are present in the basic mathematics. Pick a node in the network at random, and look at its neighbours: what would you expect *their* degrees to be? It turns out that the degrees of the neighbours of a node chosen at random tend to be greater than that of the node itself. This is because there are more opportunities to connect to a node that has high degree than to one with low degree. In a social setting this means that your friends are typically more popular than you are: they, on average, have more friends than average. This is true of any node chosen at random – and so, paradoxically, while your friends are on average more popular than you are, *their* friends are also on average more popular than

[11] Duncan Watts. *Small worlds*. Princeton Studies in Complexity. Princeton University Press, 1999

[12] Duncan Watts and Steven Strogatz. Collective dynamics of 'small-world' networks. *Nature*, 393:440–442, 1998

"Celebrity" is perhaps more suggestive of what's going on here.

[13] Duncan Watts. *Small worlds*. Princeton Studies in Complexity. Princeton University Press, 1999

them. Clearly this can't be true of everyone in the same network, and is another exmaple of how averaging can mask important detail.

Then there's the issue of randomness. One thing that's obvious about friendship networks is that they tend *not* to be random. If you have two friends, they are *likely* to be friends of each other – although not *necessarily*, as people often have disjoint sub-sets of friends. Mathematically this manifests itself as **clusters** in the network that are more highly connected that would be expected in a randomly-connected network: in fact it's breathtakingly unlikely for such structures to appear in a randomly-constructed network. Handling this clustering is mathematically very challenging, and forms one of the frontiers of current research [14]. Better models will improve the way in which we analyse social networks and improve our understansing of the processes (like diseases) that operate over them.

Powerlaw networks

So contact networks have some people who have massively more contacts than others, or than the average. This is taken to an extreme on social media, where a relatively small number of public and celebrity figures have *millions* of "friends". Even though this notion of "friendship" is different to "real" friendship, we see similar effects in physical contact networks: the networks that capture how people interact in the real world. This happens at an individual social level, where some people are natural (or enforced) recluses while others are social butterflies. It also happens through factors like work, where some people – postal workers, shop cashiers, bus drivers, teachers – interact with far more people, and far more closely, than do those in other jobs.

[14] Peter Mann, John Mitchell, V. Anne Smith, and Simon Dobson. Percolation in random graphs with higher-order clustering. Technical Report arXiv:2006.06744, arXiv, 2020

What degree distribution do such networks have? They often follow a power law, where the probability of a node having a particular degree. $p_k \propto k^{-\alpha}$ for some power $\alpha > 0$. These **powerlaw networks** [15] describe the structures of networks in a bewildering range of applications: most famously, they describe both the structure of the underlying engineering of the internet and numbers of links to web pages [16]. These networks are also called **BA networks** after their discoverers, and **scale-free** networks because their large-scale and small-scale structures look the same.

Power-law networks are not *quite* right for contact networks, though, because they can create nodes with really, *really* high degree: too high to appear in human social situations. A variation on the idea was studied by Newman, Watts, and Strogatz [17] and dounf to be a better fit. In these networks the power-law degree distribution is "cut off" before it can get too large, essentially setting a ceiling on the number of contacts an individual can have. Unsurprisingly, these networks are known as **powerlaw with cutoff networks**.

Building a contact network

Building a contact network means constructing a network where the nodes have the right degree distribution. In other words, the nodes in the network having degree k appear in the fraction predicted by the degree distribution.

When we constructed an ER network we described an algorithm that, when followed, produced a network with the desired distribution. We need a different algorithm to handle different topologies. It turns out that there is a very general algorithm, called the **configuration model**, that can construct a random network with *any* degree distribution [18].

To build a network of size N the configuration model takes a list of N numbers, each describing the degree of a node. It creates nodes with these degrees and wires their edges together

[15] Réka Albert and Albert-László Barabási. Statistical mechanics of complex networks. *Reviews of Modern Physics*, 74:47–97, January 2002

[16] Soon-Hyung Yook, Hawoong Jeong, and Albert-László Barabási. Modelling the Internet's large-scale topology. *Proceedings of the National Academy of Sciences*, 99(21), October 2002

[17] M.E.J. Newman, Duncan Watts, and Steven Strogatz. Random graph models of social networks. *Proceedings of the National Academy of Sciences*, 19, 2002

[18] Michael Molloy and Bruce Reed. A critical point for random graphs with a given degree sequence. *Random Structures and Algorithms*, 6(2–3), March–May 1995

randomly. If we can create the degree sequence we want from a degree distribution, we can use the configuration model to build a random network with nodes having those degrees.

We define a function p() that, given a degree k, returns the probability p_k of a node with that degree appearing in the network. We then define another function to which we provide this function along with the number of nodes we want, and which creates the random network. It repeatedly picks a random degree and then picks a random number betwen 0 and 1. If this second number is less than the probability of a node with that degree occurring, it adds the degree to the sequence; otrherwise it repeats the process for another degree. This continues until we have N node degrees, whih we can then pass to the configuration model to wire together.

```python
def generateFrom(N, p, maxdeg=100):
    # construct degrees according to the distribution given
    # by the model function
    rng = numpy.random.default_rng()
    ns = []
    t = 0
    for i in range(N):
        while True:
            # draw a random degree
            k = rng.integers(1, maxdeg)

            # do we include a node with this degree?
            if rng.random() < p(k):
                # yes, add it to the sequence; otherwise,
                # draw again
                ns.append(k)
                t += k
                break

    # the final sequence of degrees has to sum to an even
    # number, as each edge has two endpoints
    # if the sequence is odd, remove an element and draw
    # another from the distribution, repeating until the
    # overall sequence is even
    while t % 2 != 0:
```

(continues on next page)

(continued from previous page)

```
        # pick a node at random
        i = rng.integers(0, len(ns) - 1)

        # remove it from the sequence and from the total
        t -= ns[i]
        del ns[i]

        # choose a new node to replace the one we removed
        while True:
            # draw a new degree from the distribution
            k = rng.integers(1, maxdeg)

            # do we include a node with this degree?
            if rng.random() < p(k):
                # yes, add it to the sequence; otherwise,
                # draw again
                ns.append(k)
                t += k
                break

    # populate the network using the configuration
    # model with the given degree distribution
    g = networkx.configuration_model(ns,
                            create_using=networkx.
 Graph())
    return g
```

We now need to describe the powerlaw-with-cutoff degree distribution. Mathematically the probability of encountering a node of degree k under this distribution is given by

$$p_k \propto k^{-\alpha} e^{-k/\kappa}$$

Since the distribution is described by two parameters – the exponent α and the cutoff κ – we define a function that takes these two parameters and returns a function that returns p_k for any degree k.

```
def makePowerlawWithCutoff(alpha, cutoff):
    C = 1.0 / mpmath.polylog(alpha, numpy.exp(-1.0 / cutoff))
    def p(k):
```

(continues on next page)

The number C in this function is just a normalising constant needed to make the probabilities for the different degrees sum to 1 so that they form a valid probability distribution.

(continued from previous page)

```
        return (pow((k + 0.0), -alpha) * numpy.exp(-(k + 0.0) /
→ cutoff)) * C
    return p
```

We can then show the degree distribution that results, by again creating a network and then plotting a histogram of the degrees of the nodes.

```
# a small sample network
N = 10000
alpha = 2
cutoff = 40

# generate the network from the parameters describing the
# degree distribution
g = generateFrom(N, makePowerlawWithCutoff(alpha, cutoff))
```

```
fig = plt.figure(figsize=(8, 8))
ax = fig.gca()

# draw the degree distribution
ks = list(dict(networkx.degree(g)).values())
ax.hist(ks, bins=max(ks))
ax.set_title('Powerlaw-with-cutoff degree distribution ($N =
→{n}, \\alpha = {e}, \\kappa = {k}$)'.format(n=N, e=alpha,
→k=cutoff), y=1.05)
ax.semilogy()
ax.set_xlabel('$k$')
ax.set_ylabel('$\\log \\, N_k$')
plt.show()
```

Powerlaw-with-cutoff degree distribution ($N = 10000, \alpha = 2, \kappa = 40$)

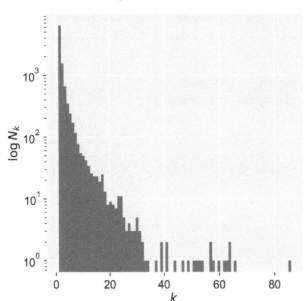

Notice that the number of nodes falls exponentially until it hits the cutoff (40), after which it becomes very sparse indeed: there are very few nodes with degrees larger than the cutoff value.

Epidemics spreading on powerlaw networks

Now that we can build a human contact network, we can again run epidemics over it to see what happens: is there an equivalent of the epidemic threshold that we saw for ER networks?

Again, we need to conduct some fairly intensive simulation.

```
lab = epyc.ClusterLab(profile='hogun',
                      notebook=epyc.JSONLabNotebook('datasets/
 threshold-plc.json', create=True))
```

We define a class that constructs random-powerlaw-with cutoff networks, essentially just importing the code we developed above into the simulator.

```
%%pxlocal

class PLCNetworkDynamics(epydemic.StochasticDynamics):

    # Experimental paramerters
    N = 'N'
    ALPHA = 'alpha'
    CUTOFF = 'cutoff'

    def __init__(self, p):
        super(PLCNetworkDynamics, self).__init__(p)

    def makePowerlawWithCutoff(self, alpha, cutoff):
        C = 1.0 / mpmath.polylog(alpha, numpy.exp(-1.0 /
cutoff))
        def p(k):
            return (pow((k + 0.0), -alpha) * numpy.exp(-(k + 0.
0) / cutoff)) * C
        return p

    def generatePLC(self, N, alpha, cutoff, maxdeg=100):
        p = self.makePowerlawWithCutoff(alpha, cutoff)
        rng = numpy.random.default_rng()
        ns = []
        t = 0
        for i in range(N):
            while True:
                k = rng.integers(1, maxdeg)
                if rng.random() < p(k):
                    ns.append(k)
                    t += k
                    break
        while t % 2 != 0:
            i = rng.integers(0, len(ns) - 1)
            t -= ns[i]
            del ns[i]
            while True:
                k = rng.integers(1, maxdeg)
                if rng.random() < p(k):
                    ns.append(k)
                    t += k
                    break
        return networkx.configuration_model(ns,
```

(continues on next page)

Epidemics spreading on powerlaw networks

(continued from previous page)

```
                                    create_
→using=networkx.Graph())

    def configure(self, params):
        super(PLCNetworkDynamics, self).configure(params)

        # build a random powerlaw-with-cutoff network
        # with the given parameters
        N = params[self.N]
        alpha = params[self.ALPHA]
        cutoff = params[self.CUTOFF]
        g = self.generatePLC(N, alpha, cutoff)
        self.setNetworkPrototype(g)
```

From this we can build a sample network.

```
N = 10000
alpha = 2
cutoff = 10
```

And then define a parameter space over which to to run experiments. We run a normal SIR process for the range of infection probabilities (values of p_{infect}).

```
# test network
lab[PLCNetworkDynamics.N] = N
lab[PLCNetworkDynamics.ALPHA] = alpha
lab[PLCNetworkDynamics.CUTOFF] = cutoff

# disease parameters
lab[epydemic.SIR.P_INFECTED] = 0.001
lab[epydemic.SIR.P_REMOVE] = 0.002
lab[epydemic.SIR.P_INFECT] = numpy.linspace(0.00001, 1.0,
                                    num=100)
```

```
m = epydemic.SIR()
e = PLCNetworkDynamics(m)
rc = lab.runExperiment(epyc.RepeatedExperiment(
                    epyc.RepeatedExperiment(e, 10),
                10))
```

Human contact networks

Much computation again ensues before we can retrieve the results.

```
df = epyc.JSONLabNotebook('datasets/threshold-plc.json').
 dataframe()
```

Plotting the size of the resulting epidemic as before then yields the folowing:

```
fig = plt.figure(figsize=(8, 8))
ax = fig.gca()

# plot the size of the removed population
cutoffs = df[PLCNetworkDynamics.CUTOFF]
pInfects = df[[kappa == cutoff for kappa in cutoffs]]
ax.plot(pInfects[epydemic.SIR.P_INFECT],
        pInfects[epydemic.SIR.REMOVED], 'r.')
ax.set_xlabel('$p_{\\mathit{infect}}$')
ax.set_ylabel('population that is...')
ax.set_title('Epidemic size vs $p_{\\mathit{infect}}$ ' + '($N
 = {n}, \\alpha = {a}, \\kappa = {k}$)'.format(n=N, a=alpha,
 k=cutoff), y=1.05)

plt.show()
```

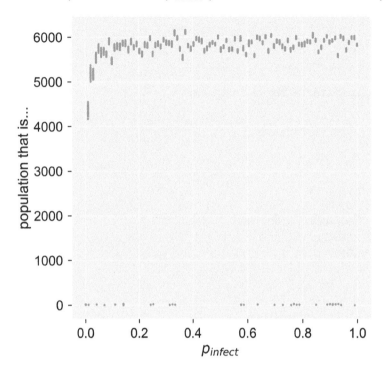

Epidemic size vs p_{infect} ($N = 10000, \alpha = 2, \kappa = 10$)

Now that's a different result! It seems that, for all values of p_{infect} we can get an epidemic, and with not a lot of variance between the repetitions. This is very much unlike the ER network case for which there was a distinct point of infection below which epidemics didn't take hold. Also different is that the size of the epidemic is relatively fixed at about 60% of the population.

If p_{infect} isn't a deciding factor in the emergence of an epidemic, might it depend on the details of the network topology? We can explore this by keeping the disease parameters the same but changing the topological parameters.

```
cutoff = 2
```

```
lab[PLCNetworkDynamics.CUTOFF] = cutoff
rc = lab.runExperiment(epyc.RepeatedExperiment(epyc.
  RepeatedExperiment(e, 10), 10))
```

```
df = epyc.JSONLabNotebook('datasets/threshold-plc.json').
 ⌐dataframe()
```

```
fig = plt.figure(figsize=(8, 8))
ax = fig.gca()

# plot the size of the removed population
cutoffs = df[PLCNetworkDynamics.CUTOFF]
pInfects = df[[kappa == cutoff for kappa in cutoffs]]
ax.plot(pInfects[epydemic.SIR.P_INFECT],
        pInfects[epydemic.SIR.REMOVED], 'r.')
ax.set_xlabel('$p_{\\mathit{infect}}$')
ax.set_ylabel('population that is...')
ax.set_title('Epidemic size vs $p_{\\mathit{infect}}$ ' + '($N_
 ⌐= {n}, \\alpha = {a}, \\kappa = {k}$)'.format(n=N, a=alpha,_
 ⌐k=cutoff), y=1.05)

plt.show()
```

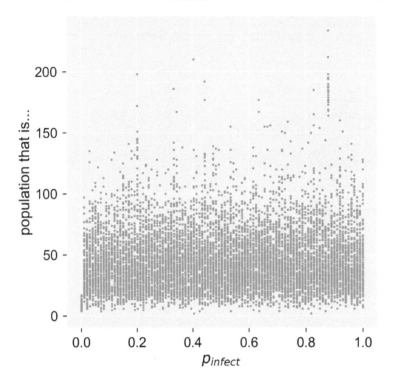

Epidemic size vs p_{infect} ($N = 10000, \alpha = 2, \kappa = 2$)

For a network with a smaller cutoff, meaning a smaller mean degree for nodes. we still get behaviour that's independent of p_{infect}. But look at the range of the y axis: instead of an epidemic through 60% of the population, we get a tiny outbreak affecting less than 5%.

A moment's thought will explain this. The cutoff is so small that the network is extremely sparse – there are very few edges between nodes – so it's difficult for the disease to spread. Another way to look at this is that a population with very few social contacts is very safe from diseases spread by contact.

The preponderance of epidemics

If we were to explore this phenomenon systematically, we'd discover that it's the value of the exponent and cutoff that control the size of the disease outbreak *not* the infectiousness of the disease. In fact there are two possible regimes for these networks, one in which epidemics *always* affect a large fraction of the population, and one in which they *never* take off [19].

From empirical studies it turns out that human contact networks tend to have an exponent of about 2, and for such networks an epidemic will break out for almost *any* value of the cutoff above 2 – and will *always* break out for powerlaw networks that don't have a cutoff. Put another way, even a small mean number of contacts won't stop an epidemic from spreading through a population, pretty much regardless of the disease's infectiousness. The reason is that the "hubs" of highly connected individuals, if they are infected, become "super-spreaders" who disseminate the epidemic widely.

This is a significant result. On the one hand, it's bad news: even minor diseases will be spread, driven by the characterics of the contact network itself. However, on the other hand, it suggests strategies for containment if we reduce the mean degree sufficiently, *or* if we tackle the issue of the hubs acting as super-spreaders. These ideas are the basis of both vaccination and social distancing.

[19] M.E.J. Newman, Duncan Watts, and Steven Strogatz. Random graph models of social networks. *Proceedings of the National Academy of Sciences*, 19, 2002

The network science community captures this insight with the catchphrase "powerlaw networks always percolate".

Questions for discussion

- Think about your friends and neighbours. Who are the "hubs? What makes them so?

- Rumours also spread through social networks: people pass information between each other. Could we model rumour-spreading (or "fake news") as a process over the network? Would it behave like a disease? Why? (Or why not?)

Herd immunity

Epidemics pass through populations by infecting the susceptible. In doing so they change the details of the population, leaving behind a trace of the epidemic's passing in the changed biology of those who were infected. In a real epidemic this includes the human cost of the infections and deaths that occur. But it also includes other, more epidemiological, traces such a change in the proportion of the population who remain susceptible to subsequent infection.

Immunity

By **immunity** we mean making an individual impervious to future infection by the disease. Immunity is conferred on an individual in three main ways.

The simplest way to acquire immunity is to have had the disease before. Having been exposed to (and presumably defeated) the disease pathogen, the immune system stores information about the necessary response. If exposed to the pathogen again, the immune system is able to respond more quickly by having been sensitised to the pathogen. This means that the immune response starts more quickly after exposure, with less pathogen to contend with, and often means that the individual never becomes symptomatic.

This isn't quite the same as saying that the immune individual can't be re-infected. They *are* re-infected, but defeat that infection far more efficiently than does a "normal" individual.

For some diseases, an infection confers immunity on the pre-natal children of any mothers who are infected. This is a clever piece of evolution that means that children born into the midst of an epidemic are often immune to the disease to which their mother was exposed.

The widespread use of vaccines in the modern world for serious diseases is the final way to confer immunity. A vaccine essentially just pre-sensitises a person's immune system in the same way that a pre-occurring infection would do, changing their individual susceptibility without the disadvantage of making them sick.

Many diseases pathogens can't cross the placental barrier, so the mother doesn't infect the child but can still pass on her acquired immunity.

Herd immunity

If immunity is the inability of an individual to contract a disease, then **herd immunity** is the corresponding property for a population that can't undergo an epidemic of the disease. More precisely, in a herd-immune population any outbreak of the disease will tend to die out quickly without infecting a large fraction of the population.

To understand herd immunity we need to return to the initial notions we had of how an epidemic grows and persists in a population. We saw that contact trees capture the case reproduction number $\mathcal{R}$ of an ongoing epidemic. We also saw that if $\mathcal{R} \geq 1$ then the epidemic continues, as the next generation of cases is at least the same size as the previous one. If, however, $\mathcal{R}$ falls and remains below 1, then the size of the next generation is smaller than the previous one, and if this trend continues then the disease will die out.

Herd immunity occurs when $\mathcal{R} \ll 1$ so that any epidemic never gets started. More importantly, it means that if an epidemic re-starts through the disease being re-introduced, it won't get re-started. This doesn't mean that no-one ever gets infected in a herd-immune population: it's perfectly possible for people to come into contact with infected individuals from outside, and to become infected themselves if they aren't personally immune. But the disease doesn't spread from them into the rest of the population.

How does this come about? When discussing $\mathcal{R}$ we saw that it is affected by three things: the duration of infectiousness, the probability of disease transmission per contact, and the rate of contacts between infected and susceptible individuals. The first two are properties of the disease, while the second is a property of the environment in which it finds itself. A herd-immune population is one in which the number of contacts between susceptible and infected individuals is too low to sustain an outbreak, because there are too few susceptibles around. Essentially herd immunity fragments the topology of the contact network to reduce the value of $\mathcal{R}$ below the critical threshold of 1.

Epidemics on a residual network

We can model the effects of herd immunity by using the idea of a disease *repeatedly* being introduced to the *same* contact network. We let the disease run through the population, and then note that, for SIR infections, anyone who has been removed from the population cannot be re-infected, and indeed takes no further part in the disease dynamics. We are left with a **residual network** into which we re-introduce the disease by seeding it with new infected individuals, and see what happens.

There are other disease models such as SIS in which people become susceptible again after infection, and these can be used to study **endemic** diseases that remain active over a long time .
Saray Shai and Simon Dobson. Coupled adaptive complex networks. *Physical Review E*, 87(4), April 2013

The important thing to notice is that the second epidemic is caused by the re-introduction of the *same* disease, with the same infectiousness and period of infection. Will this instance of the disease spread? – only if the residual network is such that the disease can take hold in it. If the first epidemic caused enough nodes to be removed, then this may prevent a second epidemic in the same population (or, more accurately, in a large sub-set of the fraction of the population who weren't infected the first time).

This is another way to think about herd immunity. By removing nodes from the population it changes its topology so that disease propagation is no longer possible, or at least occurs at a radically smaller level. Any subsequent outbreaks are in some sense "squashed by the topology" even though the biology of the situation is unchanged.

For simplicity let's return to ER networks. (The same arguments work perfectly well on powerlaw networks too.) We create a small network and run an SIR epidemic over it, choosing disease parameters that we know will create an epidemic.

```
N = 5000
kmean = 20

T = 5000

pInfected = 0.01
pInfect = 0.0002    # above the epidemic threshold
pRemove = 0.002
```

```
g = networkx.gnp_random_graph(N, (kmean + 0.0) / N)
```

```
param = dict()
param[epydemic.SIR.P_INFECTED] = pInfected
param[epydemic.SIR.P_INFECT] = pInfect
param[epydemic.SIR.P_REMOVE] = pRemove
param[epydemic.Monitor.DELTA] = T / 50
```

```
m1 = MonitoredSIR()
e1 = epydemic.StochasticDynamics(m1, g)
rc1 = e1.set(param).run()
```

We can now see how many nodes were infected in the course of the epidemic (the size of the **R** compartment) and how many escaped infection and remain susceptible.

```
print('Remaining susceptible {s}, removed {r}'.format(s=len(m1.
↪compartment(epydemic.SIR.SUSCEPTIBLE)), r=len(m1.
↪compartment(epydemic.SIR.REMOVED))))
```

```
Remaining susceptible 1376, removed 3624
```

Quite a large epidemic, but one that left a substantial number uninfected. We now construct the residual network by deleting all the nodes who are (or have been) infected, leaving the susceptibles. We don't touch the edges between the nodes that remain.

```
h = m1.network().copy()
h.remove_nodes_from(m1.compartment(epydemic.SIR.INFECTED))
h.remove_nodes_from(m1.compartment(epydemic.SIR.REMOVED))
```

As a sanity check, the number of nodes in the residual network should match the number of susceptible nodes who were left after the first epidemic.

```
print('Order of residual network {o}'.format(o=h.order()))
```

```
Order of residual network 1376
```

We now run the *same* disease on this network without touching the experimental parameters.

```
m2 = MonitoredSIR()
e2 = epydemic.StochasticDynamics(m2, h)
rc2 = e2.set(param).run()
```

What is the result? We can plot the progress of the two epidemics side by side: the "main" epidemic and the secondary infection on the residual network.

```
(fig, axs) = plt.subplots(1, 2, sharey=True, figsize=(12, 6))

# plot the first epidemic
ax = axs[0]
timeseries1 = rc1[epyc.Experiment.RESULTS][epydemic.Monitor.
 ↪TIMESERIES]
ts1 = timeseries1[epydemic.Monitor.OBSERVATIONS]
ss1 = timeseries1[epydemic.SIR.SUSCEPTIBLE]
is1 = timeseries1[epydemic.SIR.INFECTED]
rs1 = timeseries1[epydemic.SIR.REMOVED]
ax.plot(ts1, ss1, 'r-', label='susceptible')
ax.plot(ts1, is1, 'g-', label='infected')
```

(continues on next page)

(continued from previous page)

```
ax.plot(ts1, rs1, 'k-', label='removed')
ax.set_xlabel('$t$')
ax.set_ylabel('population that is...')
ax.set_title('First epidemic')
ax.legend(loc='center right')

# plot the second epidemic on the residual network
ax = axs[1]
timeseries2 = rc2[epyc.Experiment.RESULTS][epydemic.Monitor.
 ↪TIMESERIES]
ts2 = timeseries2[epydemic.Monitor.OBSERVATIONS]
ss2 = timeseries2[epydemic.SIR.SUSCEPTIBLE]
is2 = timeseries2[epydemic.SIR.INFECTED]
ax.plot(ts2, ss2, 'r-', label='susceptible')
ax.plot(ts2, is2, 'g-', label='infected')
ax.set_xlabel('$t$')
ax.set_title('Second epidemic')
ax.legend(loc='center right')

# fine-time the figure
plt.suptitle('Progress of two epidemics on the same contact␣
↪network', y=1.05)
axs[0].set_ylabel('population that is...')

_ = plt.show()
```

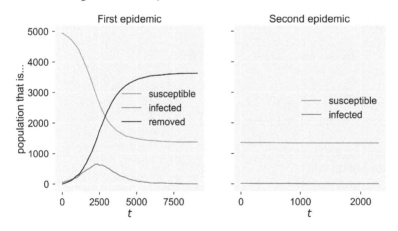

The first epidemic happens as we would expect: a burst of

---

infections followed by a dying-away. But the second epidemic looks as though nothing happens. We can check by looking at the final compartment sizes.

```
print('Remaining susceptible {s}, removed {r}'.format(s=len(m2.
→compartment(epydemic.SIR.SUSCEPTIBLE)), r=len(m2.
→compartment(epydemic.SIR.REMOVED)))))
```

```
Remaining susceptible 1340, removed 36
```

So the same disease barely affected any nodes, despite being re-introduced.

Why is this? The first epidemic changed the topology of the network. Specifically it reduced the mean degree of nodes because so many of the nodes were removed. In doing so it reduced the disease's opportunities to spread, effectively reducing $\mathcal{R}$ below the critical threshold.

```
print('Mean degree of initial network {kmean}'.
→format(kmean=kmean))
print('Mean degree of residual network {kmean:.2f}'.
→format(kmean=numpy.mean(list(dict(h.degree()).values()))))
```

```
Mean degree of initial network 20
Mean degree of residual network 5.50
```

We can show this graphically – if less scientifically usefully – by plotting the progress of the disease through the network.

```
(fig,axs) = plt.subplots(1, 3, figsize=(12, 5))

# colours fgor compartments
colours = dict()
colours[epydemic.SIR.SUSCEPTIBLE] = 'red'
colours[epydemic.SIR.INFECTED] = 'green'
colours[epydemic.SIR.REMOVED] = 'black'

# plot the final network of the first epidemic,
# colouring for compartment
ax = axs[0]
```

(continues on next page)

(continued from previous page)

```
final = m1.network()
pos1 = networkx.drawing.layout.random_layout(final)
ncs = [ colours[m1.getCompartment(n)] for n in final.nodes() ]
networkx.draw_networkx(final, pos=pos1, ax=ax,
                       node_color=ncs, node_size=5,
                       with_labels=False, edgelist=[])
ax.axis('off')
ax.set_title('After first epidemic')

# plot residual network for the second epidemic
ax = axs[1]
final = m2.network()
pos2 = { n: pos1[n] for n in pos1.keys() if n in final.nodes()
↪}
networkx.draw_networkx(final, pos=pos2, ax=ax,
                       node_color=colours[epydemic.SIR.
↪SUSCEPTIBLE],
                       node_size=5, with_labels=False,
↪edgelist=[])
ax.axis('off')
ax.set_title('Residual susceptibles')

# plot the final network of the second epidemic
ax = axs[2]
ncs = [ colours[m2.getCompartment(n)] for n in final.nodes() ]
networkx.draw_networkx(final, pos=pos2, ax=ax,
                       node_color=ncs, node_size=5,
                       with_labels=False, edgelist=[])
ax.axis('off')
ax.set_title('After second epidemic')

# fine-tune figure
plt.suptitle('Progress of two epidemics', y=1.05)

# the figure we've created is large -- very large,
# actually -- because of the large network. Since we
# don't want to create a large notebook, we generate
# and save the # file without displaying it and then
# re-load the saved image
plt.savefig('herd-finals.png', dpi=300, bbox_inches='tight')
plt.close(fig)
```

Progress of two epidemics

After first epidemic   Residual susceptibles   After second epidemic

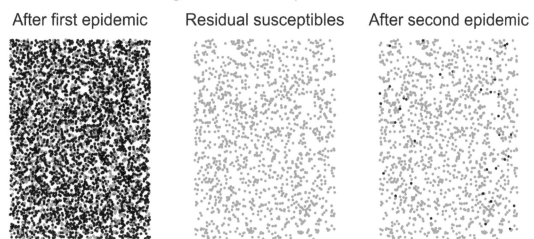

In the left-hand panel we have the network after the first epidemic, with black nodes being those that have been infected. In the middle panel we remove these nodes, leaving only the residual susceptibles. (We've not drawn the edges for reasons of scale.) In the right-hand panel we show the network after the second epidemic – look carefully to find the nodes that were infected! The visual first impression is what's important, though: after the first epidemic the network had been mostly infected, but after the second it was largely untouched despite the fact that the same disease was introduced both times. The population has been rendered herd-immune by its first brush with the disease. Even though some people were infected, the disease never took hold a second time.

The complexities of immunity

This description makes things sound simple. Infecting the population once means that they can't, as a body, be infected again, and so the risks of subsequent disease outbreaks are minimised.

Not quite. There are more things we need to consider.

Firstly, and most importantly, gaining herd immunity through infection means that a lot of people have to become sick. Depending on the disease, that can result in a lot of misery and a lot of death. We glossed-over the difference between these two factors in using SIR as our disease model, but we need to remember that "removed" (in the SIR sense) includes both those who recovered and those who died – neither of whom, in this simple model, take any further part in this or future epidemics.

While the difference between being recovered and being dead therefore doesn't matter mathematically, it matters a lot to the individuals concerned – or rather, it matters to those who survive. If a disease with even a low death rate infects 60% of a population that still potentially means a *lot* of deaths.

Secondly, a further assumption of SIR is that immunity is a binary event: one is *either* susceptible *or* removed, and if susceptible one is *entirely* susceptible and if removed one is *completely* removed. If one becomes infected, one switches instantaneously between these two classes. These assumptions aren't an accurate model of real diseases.

In many diseases, infection by the disease confers only **partial immunity** to further infection. Essentially this decreases an individual's own personal probability p_{infect}, making them less likely to be infected at subsequent encounters.

In other diseases, infection confers **temporary immunity** so that an individual's p_{infect} changes with time, perhaps dropping to zero immediately after recovery and rising over time. The exact way in which immunity decays may be different too, perhaps rising steadily or perhaps jumping, and perhaps eventually reaching a "normal" level as though the first infection hadn't occurred. And of course one can always have the case of **temporary partial immunity** that combines the features of both.

To these complexities we also need to add uncertainty. In an epidemic of a new disease we almost certainly *don't know* what, if any, immunity infection confers. This implies that we don't know whether a recurrence of the disease will result in another epidemic or not.

All this means that achieving herd immunity isn't a viable strategy for managing new diseases with large potential epidemic sizes, even if they're known (or assumed) to have relatively low mortality rates. A tiny fraction of a huge number can still be considerable. Fortunately herd immunity is not the only management strategy we have available to us.

Questions for discussion

- How would you work out whether a particular disease conferred full immunity, or only partial immunity?

- Is partial immunity any help in managing a disease? – it still leaves people at risk after infection

Changing individual susceptibility

We now turn to countermeasures that we can take to reduce the size of an epidemic.

There are several ways we can approach this. In this chapter we'll look at ways in which we can change an individual's response to potential infection. By making individuals less likely to be infected, we reduce the chances that an encounter will result in secondary infection and therefor reduce the chance of the disease spreading widely. We'll see that it matters *how many* individuals' susceptibility we modify, and often *which individuals*.

(In a later chapter we'll look at an alternative approach which leaves individual susceptibilities alone but changes the topology of encounters at the population level.)

Vaccination changes susceptibility at a **biological** level, by changing an individual's immune response, and in this chapter we'll talk about the ways in which vaccines affect epidemic spreading in a population. But it's important to remember that the same effect can be achieved at a **physical** level, with no vaccine and in fact no biological interventions at all, as we'll see later. From the perspective of epidemic spreading both biological and physical approaches behave in largely the same way.

Vaccines

For most of history we have been unable to affect the progress of diseases by biological means. Instead, we've been limited to using topology – isolation and quarantine – to reduce the spread of a disease, or slow down its progress. For many diseases these approaches were ineffective given the dynamics of the disease and the conditions of daily life for the majority of the population, and even being sufficiently rich to lock oneself away was not guaranteed to spare one from infection.

Edgar Allan Poe's short story *The Masque of the Red Death* fictionalises the ineffectiveness of this strategy, especially when faced with a supernatural opponent.

This changed at the turn of the nineteenth century with the introduction of **vaccines**. Vaccination was first tried at scale by Sir Edward Jenner, who realised the similarities between smallpox – a ravaging disease and a cause of immense suffering – and cowpox, a far milder complaint commonly encountered in milkmaids who picked it up from cattle. This proved to be the first in a long line of innovations that have now erradicated smallpox entirely.

Vaccines work by priming a person's immune system so that, if they are later infected, they already have the immunological machinery needed to fight the pathogen off. Critically, this reduces the time between infection happening and the immune response starting, meaning that there is less pathogen to fight off and therefore a better chance of preventing the infection taking hold in that individual. Sometimes this can be so effective that the individual is unaware they were even infected; more commonly they suffer a milder version of the disease, with less severe symptoms from which they recover more quickly.

There are lots of ways to build a vaccine. One can do as Jenner did and use a **mild variant** of the disease one is interested in. One can take the actual disease and produce a **denatured** version that cannot cause infection but does nevertheless prime the immune system. Modern vaccines are often even more specific than this, identifying some of the surface proteins that characterise the pathogen and introducing only them as a primer.

Immunology is an immense subject, but fortunately we don't need to understand its mechanics – how it works in *individuals* – to understand its epidemiology – how it works in *populations*. In fact, as we'll see, we don't need a vaccine in order to still get the *effects* of vaccination.

Epidemics on human contact networks

Let's revisit human contact networks as a substrate for an epidemic. Such a contact network resembles a powerlaw-with-cutoff topology rather than the "normal" topology of an ER network: there are nodes that have degrees (contacts) substantially larger than the mean of the network overall. We made the point that such networks are very good at spreading diseases.

How good? Human contact networks have different cutoffs, the point at which the probability of having nodes with higher degrees reduces dramatically. We can explore what this means by picking the dynamics of a disease and varying the cutoff to see how the *same* disease propagates on networks with *different* topologies.

```
# network parameters
N = 10000
alpha = 2

# simulation time
T = 1000

# disease dynamic parameters
pInfected = 0.001
pInfect = 0.01
pRemove = 0.002
```

```
# set up the experiment
lab = epyc.Lab()
lab[epydemic.SIR.P_INFECTED] = pInfected
lab[epydemic.SIR.P_INFECT] = pInfect
```

(continues on next page)

(continued from previous page)

```
lab[epydemic.SIR.P_REMOVE] = pRemove
lab[PLCNetworkDynamics.N] = N
lab[PLCNetworkDynamics.ALPHA] = alpha
lab[PLCNetworkDynamics.CUTOFF] = numpy.linspace(10, 80,
                                                num=4)
lab[epydemic.Monitor.DELTA] = T / 50

# perform one monitoried epidemic
m = MonitoredSIR()
e = PLCNetworkDynamics(m)
lab.runExperiment(e)
```

Plotting the results for the different cutoff values yields the following.

```
df = lab.dataframe()
cutoffs = df[PLCNetworkDynamics.CUTOFF].unique()

(fig, axs) = plt.subplots(2, 2, sharex=True, sharey=True,
                          figsize=(10, 10))

for (ax, cutoff) in [ (axs[0][0], cutoffs[0]),
                      (axs[0][1], cutoffs[1]),
                      (axs[1][0], cutoffs[2]),
                      (axs[1][1], cutoffs[3]) ]:
    rc = df[df[PLCNetworkDynamics.CUTOFF] == cutoff]
    timeseries = rc[MonitoredSIR.TIMESERIES].iloc[0]
    ts = timeseries[MonitoredSIR.OBSERVATIONS]
    sss = timeseries[epydemic.SIR.SUSCEPTIBLE]
    iss = timeseries[epydemic.SIR.INFECTED]
    rss = timeseries[epydemic.SIR.REMOVED]

    ax.plot(ts, sss, 'r.', label='suceptible')
    ax.plot(ts, iss, 'g.', label='infected')
    #ax.plot(ts, rss, 'ks', label='removed')

    ax.set_title('$\\kappa = {kappa:.0f}$'.
  format(kappa=cutoff))
    ax.set_xlim([0, T])
    ax.set_ylim([0, N])
    ax.legend(loc='upper right')
```

(continues on next page)

(continued from previous page)

```
# fine-tune the diagram
plt.suptitle('SIR over powerlaw networks for different cutoffs␣
↪($N = {n}, \\alpha={a}$)'.format(n=N, a=alpha))
for y in range(2):
    axs[y][0].set_ylabel('population that is...')
for x in range(2):
    axs[1][x].set_xlabel('$t$')

plt.show()
```

SIR over powerlaw networks for different cutoffs ($N = 10000, \alpha = 2$)

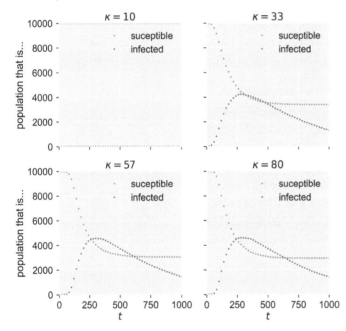

This is telling us that networks with a small maximum number of contacts ($\kappa = 10$) have relative small epidemics that appear quite slowly: the "peak" of the infections occurs farther into the outbreak. As we increase κ we see larger epidemics happening faster (closer to the start of the outbreak), until the results seem to stabilise and not change much as we continue to increase κ: a maximum of about 30 contacts seems to be enough to infect about half the popuation at the peak.

Vaccination in SIR

What does vaccination look like in the SIR model? A vaccinated individual is one who cannot catch the disease. In model terms it means that an individual who exhibits that characteristics of having already had the disease, and having been "removed" into the **R** compartment. In fact this is what's happening biologically as well: a vaccinated individual has been exposed to a substance that renders them the same *as if* they'd had the disease, without actually requiring them to *have had* it. The effect we're looking for is herd immunity, where there are insufficient susceptible individuals in a population to let the disease establish itelf. But critically we're looking for herd immunity *without having the disease pass through the population first*, with all the suffering and (possibly) death that this might entail.

We could model vaccination using a new compartment, leading to a model that might be called **SIVR** capturing the vaccinated individuals **V**. But in conditions of total vaccinated immunity the **V** individuals will behave identically to the **R** individuals, so we may as well simply treat them identically too. (If we were wanting to explore partial immunity through vaccination then SIVR would let us have, for example, different values of p_{infect} depending on whether it's an **S** or a **V** individual being potentially infected: **V** becomes a halfway-house between **S** (fully susceptible) and **R** (fully removed).

We've obviously simplified this, as anyone who's caught a disease for which they've been vaccinated will know. Vaccination doesn't always give full immunity against infection.

Vaccinating the population at random

Most vaccines are applied broadly to a population, typically in childhood for a range of common diseases which most people will face. Ideally everyone is vaccinated; in practice some are missed for various reasons, in some the vaccine will not "take", some must avoid it for unrelated medical reasons, and so forth.

We could try to model the ways in which this process happens in detail, but the overall effect is very similar to the case where we

For many years seasonal influenza vaccines were grown in chicken eggs, meaning that they were unsuitable for vegans and anyone with a dairy allergy. Modern flu vaccines aren't created this way.

take a population and randomly vaccinate some percentage of the individuals before starting the infection. Since this is SIR, this means that we randomly assign some fraction $p_{vaccinated}$ of nodes to the **R** compartment.

```python
class MonitoredVaccinatedSIR(epydemic.SIR, epydemic.Monitor):

    P_VACCINATED = 'pVaccinated'    #: Probability that an
                                    # individual is initially␣
␣removed.

    def __init__(self):
        super(MonitoredVaccinatedSIR, self).__init__()

    def build(self, params):
        '''Build the observation process.

        :param params: the experimental parameters'''
        super(MonitoredVaccinatedSIR, self).build(params)

        # change the initial compartment probabilities to␣
␣vaccinate (remove) some fraction
        pInfected = params[epydemic.SIR.P_INFECTED]
        pVaccinated = params[self.P_VACCINATED]
        self.changeCompartmentInitialOccupancy(epydemic.SIR.
␣INFECTED, pInfected)
        self.changeCompartmentInitialOccupancy(epydemic.SIR.
␣REMOVED, pVaccinated)
        self.changeCompartmentInitialOccupancy(epydemic.SIR.
␣SUSCEPTIBLE, 1.0 - pInfected - pVaccinated)

        # also monitor other compartments
        self.trackNodesInCompartment(epydemic.SIR.SUSCEPTIBLE)
        self.trackNodesInCompartment(epydemic.SIR.REMOVED)
```

We can choose any number we like for $p_{vaccinated}$, with 60% being a typical target for immunisation campaigns.

```python
pVaccinated = 0.6
```

Leaving all other experimental parameters the same from above, let's choose a value of $\kappa = 57$ as a cutoff that we saw created an epidemic in a unvaccinated population, and run an experiment where we first vaccinate (remove) a fraction of nodes at random.

```
lab[MonitoredVaccinatedSIR.P_VACCINATED] = pVaccinated
lab[PLCNetworkDynamics.CUTOFF] = 57

m = MonitoredVaccinatedSIR()
e = PLCNetworkDynamics(m)
lab.runExperiment(e)

df = lab.dataframe()
```

We can then see the progress of the *same* epidemic on the *same* network topology, but in the presence of an effective vaccine applied to a fraction of the population.

```
fig = plt.figure(figsize=(8, 8))
ax = fig.gca()

rc = df[df[MonitoredVaccinatedSIR.P_VACCINATED] == 0.6]
results = rc.iloc[0]
timeseries = results[epydemic.Monitor.TIMESERIES]
ts = timeseries[MonitoredVaccinatedSIR.OBSERVATIONS]
sss = timeseries[epydemic.SIR.SUSCEPTIBLE]
iss = timeseries[epydemic.SIR.INFECTED]
rss = timeseries[epydemic.SIR.REMOVED]
ax.plot(ts, sss, 'r.', label='suceptible')
ax.plot(ts, iss, 'g.', label='infected')
#ax.plot(ts, rss, 'ks', label='removed')

ax.set_xlim([0, T])
ax.set_xlabel('$t$')
ax.set_ylim([0, N * (1.0 - pVaccinated - pInfected)])
ax.set_ylabel('population that is...')
ax.set_title('SIR epidemic in the presence of {v:.0f}%
 ↪vaccination ($\\kappa = {k}$)'.
 ↪format(v=results[MonitoredVaccinatedSIR.P_VACCINATED] * 100,
 ↪k=results[PLCNetworkDynamics.CUTOFF]), y=1.05)
ax.legend(loc='upper right')

plt.show()
```

SIR epidemic in the presence of 60% vaccination ($\kappa = 57.0$)

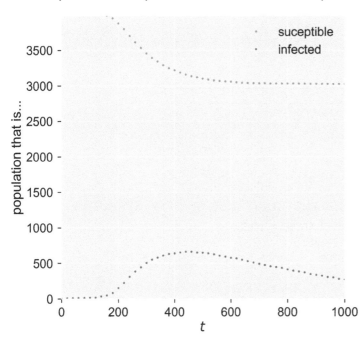

Comparing this to the figure above shows quite a dramatic reduction in the outbreak size.

But wait! – there might be a problem Look at the y-axis in this graph. Notice that the maximum susceptible population is about 4000, even though the network has 10000 nodes. A moment's thought shows why: we modelled vaccination as being pre-emptively removed, leaving fewer susceptibles. Could it be that this result is what we'd *expect* on a smaller network? In other words, is there a size effect coming into play as we move from 10000 down to 4000 individuals?

We should be careful and check this possibility. We can do so by working out the size of the unvaccinated population and creating a network with the same topology of this size, and then running our epidemic over it.

```
Nsmall = int(N * (1.0 - pVaccinated - pInfected))
lab[PLCNetworkDynamics.N] = Nsmall
```

(continues on next page)

Vaccinating the population at random

(continued from previous page)

```
m = MonitoredSIR()
e = PLCNetworkDynamics(m)
lab.runExperiment(e)
df = lab.dataframe()
```

```
fig = plt.figure(figsize=(8, 8))
ax = fig.gca()

# plot epidemic on unvaccinated network
rc = df[df[PLCNetworkDynamics.N] == Nsmall]
results = rc.iloc[0]
timeseries = results[epydemic.Monitor.TIMESERIES]
ts = timeseries[MonitoredVaccinatedSIR.OBSERVATIONS]
sss = timeseries[epydemic.SIR.SUSCEPTIBLE]
iss = timeseries[epydemic.SIR.INFECTED]
rss = timeseries[epydemic.SIR.REMOVED]
ax.plot(ts, sss, 'r.', label='suceptible (no vaccination)')
ax.plot(ts, iss, 'g.', label='infected (no vaccination)')
#ax.plot(ts, rss, 'ks', label='removed')

# plot results on same-sized network reduced in
# size by vaccination
rc = df[df[MonitoredVaccinatedSIR.P_VACCINATED] == 0.6]
results = rc.iloc[0]
timeseries = results[epydemic.Monitor.TIMESERIES]
ts = timeseries[MonitoredVaccinatedSIR.OBSERVATIONS]
sss = timeseries[epydemic.SIR.SUSCEPTIBLE]
iss = timeseries[epydemic.SIR.INFECTED]
rss = timeseries[epydemic.SIR.REMOVED]
ax.plot(ts, sss, 'ro', label='suceptible (post vaccination)')
ax.plot(ts, iss, 'go', label='infected (post vaccination)')
#ax.plot(ts, rss, 'ks', label='removed')
ax.set_xlim([0, T])
ax.set_xlabel('$t$')
ax.set_ylim([0, Nsmall])
ax.set_ylabel('population that is...')
ax.set_title('SIR epidemic with and without vaccination ($N =
↪{n}, \\kappa = {k}$'.format(n=Nsmall,␣
↪k=results[PLCNetworkDynamics.CUTOFF]), y=1.05)
ax.legend(loc='center right')
```

(continues on next page)

(continued from previous page)

```
plt.show()
```

SIR epidemic with and without vaccination ($N = 3990, \kappa = 57.0$)

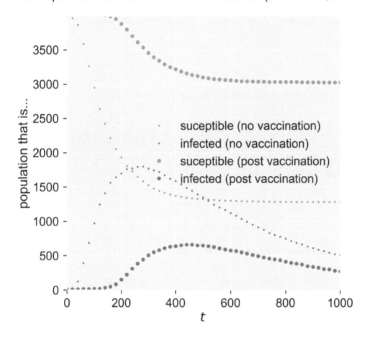

The first thing to see is that the two graphs are different:
it's not *just* the size of the network that affects things. In the
small-but-unvaccinated network we see a larger epidemic; in the
vaccinated network we see a much smaller and slower outbreak.
What is different between the two cases, since the networks are
the same size?

A moment's thought may suggest the answer. We've created
two networks with the same topology, one where a fraction of
nodes are removed by vaccination, and one where a number of
nodes really had been removed (or rather, were never present in
the network in the first place). Both networks have high-degree
nodes, as we'd expect for powerlaw-with-cutoff networks. But in
the latter (vaccinated) case, some of those high-degree nodes will
have been vaccinated and so are not able to spread the disease.

And since the disease spreads through contact between **S** and **I** nodes, we lose the opportunity to infect a high-degree node that could act as super-spreaders able to infect a large number of nodes. And that reduction in super-spreading is enough to change the dynamics of the disease.

How super are super-spreaders?

Let's look at some numbers. Firstly, how many contacts does the most highly-connected node have?

```
g = m.network()
ks = sorted(list(dict(networkx.degree(g)).values()))
print('Maximum degree = {kmax}'.format(kmax=max(ks)))
```

```
Maximum degree = 62
```

That's a high number. What about the number of contacts for an averagely-connected node?

```
print('Mean node degree = {kmean:.2f}'.format(kmean=numpy.
↪mean(ks)))
```

```
Mean node degree = 2.59
```

Very different, and it's this feature that differentiates a human contact network from an ER network: the existence of nodes with degrees that are much higher than the average. In fact such networks have a **long tail** of nodes with high degrees: only a small number relative to the size of the network overall, but nonetheless able to pass infection.

```
h = 10
print('Highest {h} nodes by degree {l}'.format(h=h, l=ks[-h:]))
```

```
Highest 10 nodes by degree [43, 44, 45, 46, 46, 50, 54, 54, 56,
↪ 62]
```

How important are these individuals in the spread of the disease? We can study that by excluding them from our model vaccination programme. Instead of vaccinating some fraction of the network, after vaccination we will make sure that some fraction of the highest-degree nodes are susceptible. Essentially we swap high-degree nodes for lower-degree nodes in our vaccination programme.

There are other ways we could do this too, for example by making the probability of vaccinating a node inversely proportional to its degree.

```python
class MonitoredVaccinatedLowDegreeSIR(MonitoredVaccinatedSIR):

    K_HIGH_FRACTION = 'k_high_fraction'

    def __init__(self):
        super(MonitoredVaccinatedLowDegreeSIR, self).__init__()

    def setUp(self, params):
        super(MonitoredVaccinatedLowDegreeSIR, self).
 →setUp(params)

        # look through the fraction of high-degree nodes and
        # make them susceptible again, replacing them with
        # another node chosen at random
        rng = numpy.random.default_rng()
        g = self.network()
        ns = list(g.nodes())
        h = int(len(ns) * params[self.K_HIGH_FRACTION])
        degrees = dict(networkx.degree(g))
        ks = sorted(list(degrees.values()))
        ks_high = set(ks[-h:])
        ns_high = [n for n in ns if degrees[n] in ks_high]
        for n in ns_high:
            if self.getCompartment(n) == self.REMOVED:
                # node is removed, make it susceptible again
                self.setCompartment(n, self.SUSCEPTIBLE)

                # choose another node and remove it in
                # place of the node we just forced to
                # be susceptible
                while True:
                    i = rng.integers(0, len(ns) - 1)
```

(continues on next page)

(continued from previous page)

```
                    m = ns[i]
                    if self.getCompartment(m) == self.
 SUSCEPTIBLE:
                        # found a susceptible node, remove it
                        self.setCompartment(m, self.REMOVED)
                        break
```

Running the experiment, again with the same disease parameters
and network topology as before, shows us the effects of this
failure in vaccination.

```
kHighFraction = 0.08  # highest-degree 8%

lab[MonitoredVaccinatedLowDegreeSIR.K_HIGH_FRACTION] =
 kHighFraction
lab[PLCNetworkDynamics.N] = N

m = MonitoredVaccinatedLowDegreeSIR()
e = PLCNetworkDynamics(m)
lab.runExperiment(e)
df = lab.dataframe()
```

```
fig = plt.figure(figsize=(8, 8))
ax = fig.gca()

rc = df[df[MonitoredVaccinatedLowDegreeSIR.K_HIGH_FRACTION] ==
 kHighFraction]
results = rc.iloc[0]
timeseries = results[epidemic.Monitor.TIMESERIES]
ts = timeseries[MonitoredVaccinatedSIR.OBSERVATIONS]
sss = timeseries[epydemic.SIR.SUSCEPTIBLE]
iss = timeseries[epydemic.SIR.INFECTED]
rss = timeseries[epydemic.SIR.REMOVED]
ax.plot(ts, sss, 'r.', label='suceptible')
ax.plot(ts, iss, 'g.', label='infected')
#ax.plot(ts, rss, 'ks', label='removed')

ax.set_xlim([0, T])
ax.set_xlabel('$t$')
ax.set_ylim([0, N * (1.0 - pInfected - pVaccinated) + N *
 kHighFraction])
```

(continues on next page)

(continued from previous page)

```
ax.set_ylabel('population that is...')
ax.set_title('SIR epidemic without vaccination of {khigh:.0f}%
 highest-degree nodes ($N = {n}, \\kappa = {k:.0f}$)'.
 format(khigh=kHighFraction * 100, n=N,
 k=results[PLCNetworkDynamics.CUTOFF]), y=1.05)
ax.legend(loc='upper right')

plt.show()
```

SIR epidemic without vaccination of 8% highest-degree nodes ($N = 10000, \kappa = 57$)

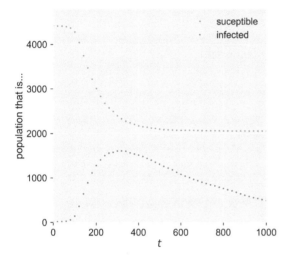

Letting a small fraction of the high-degree nodes – *i.e.*, the most connected individuals – remain susceptible changes the epidemic again, making it larger and faster. It's not only the *size* of the vaccinated population that counts: it's *who we vaccinate* (or, in this case, don't vaccinate) that really matters. Missing even a small fraction of the highly connected will radically reduce the effectiveness of a vaccination programme.

Targetted vaccination

So the existence of high-degree nodes offers an opportunity for the disease to infect far more individuals if those nodes are not protected by vaccination.

But this also offers opportunities for further countermeasures. If high-degree nodes are important in spreading the disease, what if – instead of vaccinating at random – we instead *explicitly target* those nodes that we believe are the most important in spreading the disease? That might make our programme more effective. It might also mean that we could perform a smaller, more focused, programme, where instead of vaccinating widely at random we vaccinate narrowly but in a focused, "smart" way.

We can explore this too. Rather than perform random vaccination, we instead target a specific fraction of the highest-degree nodes.

```python
class MonitoredVaccinatedHighDegreeSIR(MonitoredSIR):

    K_VACCINATED_FRACTION = 'k_vaccinated_fraction'

    def __init__(self):
        super(MonitoredVaccinatedHighDegreeSIR, self).__init__
↪()

    def setUp(self, params):
        super(MonitoredVaccinatedHighDegreeSIR, self).
↪setUp(params)

        # look for the fraction of highest-degree nodes
        # and vaccinate (remove) them
        g = self.network()
        ns = list(g.nodes())
        h = int(len(ns) * params[self.K_VACCINATED_FRACTION])
        degrees = dict(networkx.degree(g))
        ks = sorted(list(degrees.values()))
        ks_high = set(ks[-h:])
        ns_high = [n for n in ns if degrees[n] in ks_high]
        for n in ns_high:
            # remove (vaccinate) the node
            self.setCompartment(n, self.REMOVED)
```

How large a fraction do we need to target? Let's be ambitious and start small, vaccinating only 2% of nodes – thirty times fewer than before.

```
kVaccinatedFraction = 0.02     # top 2% highest-degree nodes
lab[MonitoredVaccinatedHighDegreeSIR.K_VACCINATED_FRACTION] =⌴
⌴kVaccinatedFraction

m = MonitoredVaccinatedHighDegreeSIR()
e = PLCNetworkDynamics(m)
lab.runExperiment(e)
df = lab.dataframe()
```

```
fig = plt.figure(figsize=(8, 8))
ax = fig.gca()

rc = df[df[MonitoredVaccinatedHighDegreeSIR.K_VACCINATED_
⌴FRACTION] == kVaccinatedFraction]
results = rc.iloc[0]
timeseries = results[epydemic.Monitor.TIMESERIES]
ts = timeseries[MonitoredVaccinatedSIR.OBSERVATIONS]
sss = timeseries[epydemic.SIR.SUSCEPTIBLE]
iss = timeseries[epydemic.SIR.INFECTED]
rss = timeseries[epydemic.SIR.REMOVED]
ax.plot(ts, sss, 'r.', label='suceptible')
ax.plot(ts, iss, 'g.', label='infected')
#ax.plot(ts, rss, 'ks', label='removed')

ax.set_xlim([0, T])
ax.set_xlabel('$t$')
ax.set_ylim([0, N])
ax.set_ylabel('population that is...')
ax.set_title('SIR epidemic vaccinating only the {kvac:.0f}%⌴
⌴highest-degree nodes ($N = {n}, \\kappa = {k:.0f}$)'.
⌴format(kvac=kVaccinatedFraction * 100, n=N,⌴
⌴k=results[PLCNetworkDynamics.CUTOFF]), y=1.05)
ax.legend(loc='upper right')

plt.show()
```

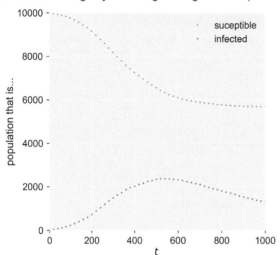

SIR epidemic vaccinating only the 2% highest-degree nodes ($N = 10000, \kappa = 57$)

That's quite amazing! With almost no-one vaccinated – 200 in a network of 10000 – we both reduce and slow the epidemic. Both these effects are important. The total number of people infected is smaller, but so too is the "ramp-up" at the start of the epidemic, which means less stress is placed on health systems dealing with the influx of sick peoiple.

When people talk of **flattening the curve**, this is the effect they're aiming at – achieved in this case through targeted vaccination of a tiny fraction of the population.

This reduction in vaccination effort makes it faster, cheaper, and more reliable – *if* we can identify and target the super-spreaders. But this might be possible, because we know that the super-spreaders are the highest-degree nodes, who are simply the ones with the most exposure to other people. In the modern world a person's contact degree is often at least partially a function of their job, and so by targeting those whose jobs bring them into contact with the most people – and especially into contact with the most *infected* people – we can create a very effective vaccination strategy and roll it out quickly.

"Vaccination" without vaccines

We said at the beginning of this chapter that immunology was an enormously complicated topic but one whose details didn't matter for population-level modelling. The experiments we conducted above have hopefully convinced you of this.

But if this is the case, then it's not vaccination that's the important feature for our purposes. Any technology *that behaves like a vaccine* preventing the infection of those we treat, will have the same effect.

What technologies might these be? An obvious example is personal protective equipment such as face masks, surgical gloves, and the like, issued to those whom we identify as being in high-contact professions such as care workers, medical workers, bus drivers, and the like – anyone who, if they were to become infected, would have the opportunity to spread the disease to a disproportionate number of others. Most importantly this doesn't require that we protect *everyone*, just that we protect *the most important* people in the contact network, whom we identify by their contact degree.

Questions for discussion

- What groups in society would you choose for targetted vaccination?

- Would you be happy *just* doing targetted vaccination, or would you want "general" vaccination too?

- If we never have a vaccine for a disease, how can we protect ourselves against it?

Asymptomatic transmission

Since we first introduced the SIR model you may have had the niggling suspicion that – while it's obviously a *simple* model of a disease – maybe it's *too* simple. We know from looking at diseases' progression (and from experience) that diseases are much more complicated than SIR suggests. In particular, many of them (the Type A diseases) have incubation periods longer than their latent periods, meaning that an individual can infect others while not showing any outward symptoms. This **asymptomatic transmission** is a problem for disease control, since it means that infectious people aren't immediately identifiable, either by people noticing their symptoms or by them noticing their own symptoms themselves.

There is of course nothing sacrosanct about SIR. It's a model: a generally useful one for studying disease phenomena, but one that we can (and should) either ditch or enrich whenever we see deficiencies or want to explore some new phenomena. One possible extension to SIR is to allow asymptomatic transmission, leading to a model that includes individuals who have been "exposed" to the disease, and who are infectious but not yet visibly symptomatic.

SEIR

SEIR is another compartmented model of disease. Like SIR, it includes compartments for individuals who are susceptible to infection, infected (and infectious), and removed from the disease by recovery or death. However, it adds a fourth compartment:

- **Exposed (E)**, representing those people who have caught the disease and can pass it on but who are not yet showing symptoms

Exposed individuals, like infected individuals, can transmit the disease to neighbouring (if we are using a networked model) susceptibles. They also transition from exposed to infected at some rate, capturing how their symptoms develop.

In the same way as we developed a mathematical model of SIR in terms of how the populations of the different compartments changed over time, we can do the same thing for SEIR. We expect to see another equation showing how the population of **E** changes, and indeed we do:

$$\Delta S = -p_{infect}\, SI - p_{infectA}\, SE$$
$$\Delta E = p_{infect}\, SI + p_{infectA}\, SE - p_{symptoms}\, E$$
$$\Delta I = p_{symptoms}\, E - p_{remove} I$$
$$\Delta R = p_{remove} I$$

What this says is that ΔS, the change in population of S, reduces S in two ways: infections coming from infected individuals at a rate that depends on the number of susceptible-infected interactions in the population – exactly as happens in SIR – but also additionally from exposed (asymptomatic) individuals at a rate (which may be different) that depends on the number of susceptible-exposed interactions. The number of exposed individuals grows at this rate, and decreases as exposed individuals develop symptoms and become infected.

Notice that we now have four compartments and four parameters:

- p_{infect}, the probability that a susceptible-infected interaction results in infection;

- $p_{infectA}$, the probability that a susceptible-exposed interaction results in infection;

- $p_{symptoms}$, the probability that an exposed individual will show symptoms; and

- p_{remove}, the probability that an infected individual will be removed.

The pros and cons of a richer model

It's reasonable to ask at this point why we don't *always* use SEIR instead of SIR, since it's clearly closer to the way a lot of real-world diseases behave. Isn't SIR *too* simple, when an only slightly more complex model is readily available in SEIR?

There are two basic arguments to make here. Firstly, SEIR has twice as many parameters as SIR: four instead of two, each of which controls some aspect of how the process works. An alternative, and very suggestive, name for the number of parameters is the number of **degrees of freedom** a model has. A model with more degrees of freedom has more "knobs you can turn" to change its behaviour. And this is both good and bad. It's good because it lets us fine-tune the model, possibly produce additional effects that a simpler model (with fewer degrees of freedom) wouldn't show. But it's bad because that means there's more work to do to fully explore all the things a model might do. If we're modelling a "real" disease, we have to collect twice as manay parameters about it. Some of these might be hard to collect: how would you go about funding $p_{infectA}$, the rate of asymptopmatic infection, when by definition asymptomatic people are hard to find?

The second argument cuts to the heart of scientific model-making. As we've seen, SIR lets us demonstrate a lot of interesting phenomena. It varies depending on the infection rate, depending on the network topology, depending on the way we apply individual countermeasures, and so forth – and we haven't finished yet! We can say a lot about diseases *in general* from SIR, even though there are lots of diseases that it can't robustly capture and for which *in detail* SEIR is better. So whether a given model is "correct" depends to a large extent on the questions we're asking.

Scientists generally prefer the simplest model that's complex enough to answer the questions they're asking. That often means minimising the number of degrees of freedom in a model, to simplify exploration and to avoid any risk that it might be "steered" in a particular direction by unfounded assumptions. It also means that a lot of detail is elided, with the danger that some of this detail may turn out to be important. This is what makes science itself into a process of continuous error and correction.

This is related to the principle of Occam's razor, which may be paraphrased as "keep things as simple as possible (but no simpler)".

Simulating SEIR

We can of course build simulations of SEIR running over a network – so let's do so.

We now have four parameters to specify instead of SIR's two: the rate $p_{infectA}$ of asymptomatic transmission (from exposed individuals to susceptibles), and the rate $p_{symptoms}$ at which symptoms show themselves. We'll explore the way in which asymptomatic transmission affects the size of the eventual outbreak. SEIR also includes an additional event when a person is **exposed** to the disease (and becomes infectious). We re-use the **infected** event as when the person becomes symptomatic.

```
lab = epyc.ClusterLab(profile='hogun',
                notebook=epyc.JSONLabNotebook('datasets/
  seir-er.json', create=True))
```

Monitoring an SEIR epidemic is essentially the same as the way we monitored SIR: we record the sizes of the compartments as the epidemic progresses.

```
%%pxlocal
```

(continues on next page)

Asymptomatic transmission

(continued from previous page)

```python
class MonitoredSEIR(epydemic.SEIR, epydemic.Monitor):

    def __init__(self):
        super(MonitoredSEIR, self).__init__()

    def build(self, params):
        '''Build the observation process.

        :param params: the experimental parameters'''
        super(MonitoredSEIR, self).build(params)

        # also monitor other compartments
        self.trackNodesInCompartment(epydemic.SEIR.SUSCEPTIBLE)
        self.trackNodesInCompartment(epydemic.SEIR.REMOVED)
```

Let's explore the outbreak on an ER network again, choosing some values for the different disease parameters and then exploring how the results vary with the value of $p_{infectA}$.

```python
# network parameters
N = 10000
kmean = 40

# SEIR disease parameters
pExposed = 0.001
pSymptoms = 0.002
pRemove = 0.002
pInfect = 0.000075
```

```python
lab[ERNetworkDynamics.N] = N
lab[ERNetworkDynamics.KMEAN] = kmean
lab[epydemic.SEIR.P_EXPOSED] = pExposed
lab[epydemic.SEIR.P_SYMPTOMS] = pSymptoms
lab[epydemic.SEIR.P_REMOVE] = pRemove
lab[epydemic.SEIR.P_INFECT_SYMPTOMATIC] = pInfect
lab[epydemic.SEIR.P_INFECT_ASYMPTOMATIC] = numpy.linspace(0.
 _00001, 0.0002, num=50)
```

```python
m = epydemic.SEIR()
e = ERNetworkDynamics(m)
```

(continues on next page)

(continued from previous page)

```
rc = lab.runExperiment(epyc.RepeatedExperiment(
                    epyc.RepeatedExperiment(e, 10),
                10))
```

After much computation, we can plot the results. We'll also show the value of "normal" infection (by symptomatic individuals) for comparison.

```
df = epyc.JSONLabNotebook('datasets/seir-er.json').dataframe()
```

```
fig = plt.figure(figsize=(8, 8))
ax = fig.gca()

# plot the size of the removed population and
# the value of symptomatic infection
ax.plot(df[epydemic.SEIR.P_INFECT_ASYMPTOMATIC],
        df[epydemic.SEIR.REMOVED], 'r.')
ax.plot([pInfect, pInfect], [0, N], 'b:')
ax.set_xlabel('$p_{\\mathit{infectA}}$')
ax.set_ylabel('population that is...')
ax.set_title('Epidemic size vs $p_{\\mathit{infectA}}$', y=1.
 ⌐05)

_ = plt.show()
```

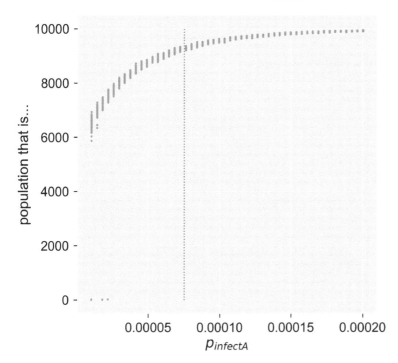

Compare this with the diagram we drew for the epidemic threshold, and you'll see that the epidemic takes off a lot earlier – which is probably what we expected, since there's more infection going on. In fact even a very small amout of early infection is enough to cause an outbreak.

```
fig = plt.figure(figsize=(8, 8))
ax = fig.gca()

# plot the size of the removed population
pInfectAs = df[[pInfect > 0.0 and pInfect < 0.00003
                for pInfect in df[epydemic.SEIR.P_INFECT_
 ASYMPTOMATIC]]]
ax.plot(pInfectAs[epydemic.SEIR.P_INFECT_ASYMPTOMATIC],
        pInfectAs[epydemic.SEIR.REMOVED], 'r.')
ax.set_xlabel('$p_{\\mathit{infectA}}$')
ax.set_ylabel('population that is...')
ax.set_title('Epidemic size vs $p_{\\mathit{infectA}}$', y=1.
 05)
```

(continues on next page)

(continued from previous page)

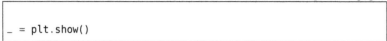

```
_ = plt.show()
```

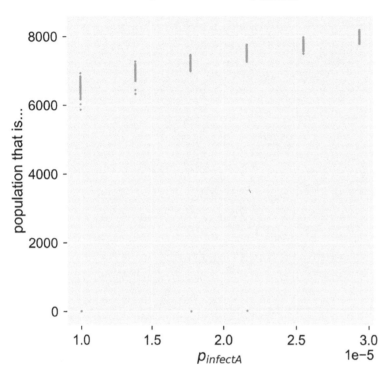

How sensitive *is* the model to asymptomatic infection? To
what extent can asymptomatic infection make a less infectious
disease behave like a more infectious disease that *doesn't* have
asymptomatic transmission? And perhaps most importantly, can
we do anything about it? It's this last question that we'll turn to
now.

Adaptive countermeasures and quarantine

We earlier discussed an approach to epidemic control that
involved targeting individual susceptibility, eliminating the

possibility of particular individuals becoming infected. This was enough to fragment the contact network and so affect the behaviour of the epidemic.

We'll now look at a completely different strategy for countermeasures. Instead of affecting individuals while leaving the network intact, we'll instead leave the individuals as they are but change the network as the epidemic spreads. That is to say, we'll change the structure of contacts – who's connected to whom – in response to the spread of the disease through the population. This leads to a family of **adaptive** countermeasures, since we take action to change the network in response to (adapting to) the process (disease) flowing through it.

The simplest and best-known adaptive control measure is **quarantine**, whereby we isolate individuals who are (or may be) infected to prevent them infecting others. A **proactive quarantine** isolates all incoming individuals for as long as it takes to pass through the expected infectious period of whatever disease they might be carrying. A **reactive or adaptive quarantine** waits until a person shows symptoms and then isolates them, which avoids detaining the uninfected but at the risk of allowing infected (and possibly infectious) people to circulate.

However it's done, the goal of quarantine is to reduce the effective $\mathcal{R}$ value of the disease such that any epidemic is contained, ideally failing to take hold or at least being smaller and less intense than would otherwise be the case.

The term "quarantine" comes from the Italian phrase for "forty days" (*quaranta giorni*). When Venice suffered an outbreak of the Black Death in the 14th century, the Venetians established a system whereby ships arriving in port had to moor off remote islands in the lagoon for forty days until they were judged to be disease-free – possibly the first modern example of effective disease control .

Sara Toth Stub. Venice's Black Death and the dawn of quarantine. *Sapiens*, April 2020

Reducing infection through partial quarantine

Let's introduce quarantine into our models. In the spirit of simplicity, we'll look first at SIR.

How does quarantine manifest itself in SIR? Infection in SIR happens when the disease passes from an infected individual to a susceptible one. Quarantine is an adaptive strategy – it happens in parallel with infection – so we'll be introducing a way of changing the network. When the disease passes to a formerly-susceptible person, we'll changes that person's connections in some way.

If this strategy was performed perfectly and immediately it would immediately stamp-out an SIR infection. Every time someone became infected, that person would be immediately and completely isolated, and so would be unable to infect anyone else. The original "seeding" of infected individuals would infect some of their neighbours, but those neighbours would then *never affect anyone else* (because they'd have no connections through which to pass the disease), and so the disease would immediately come to an end.

This clearly isn't very interesting. Nor is it very possible, other than as a theoretical best-case: in practice one would either leave infected people connected for some time before identifying and isolating them; or would only manage to isolate them from a fraction of their susceptible neighbours; or both. For our purposes we'll focus on the second option. When someone becomes infected, we immediately select some fraction of their susceptible neighbours and remove the connection to the newly-infected person. (Shai and Dobson explored this approach in a slightly more complicated scenario [20], for endemic diseases travelling through semi-isolated populations.)

[20] Saray Shai and Simon Dobson. Coupled adaptive complex networks. *Physical Review E*, 87(4), April 2013

$P_{quarantine}$ would be an alternative (and possibly better) name for this parameter.

Quarantine manifests itself as **network rewiring**: when a node becomes infected, we change the nodes to which it is connected, removing some fraction P_{rewire} of its adjacent susceptible neighbours. This naturally means that there are then fewer nodes that the newly-infected node can infect in its turn.

We introduce this into our model in two ways. Firstly, we change the behaviour of infection to include the quarantine step. Second, we define the rewiring operation over all the node's neighbours.

```
%%pxlocal

class AdaptiveSIR(MonitoredSIR):
```

(continues on next page)

(continued from previous page)

```
    P_REWIRE = 'pRewire'    #: Parameter for the probability
                            # of rewiring an SE or SI edge.


    def __init__(self):
        super(AdaptiveSIR, self).__init__()


    def build(self, params):
        super(AdaptiveSIR, self).build(params)

        # store the parameters for later
        self._pRewire = params[self.P_REWIRE]


    def quarantine(self, n):
        g = self.network()
        rng = numpy.random.default_rng()

        # run through all the neighbours of the infected node
        ms = list(g.neighbors(n))
        for m in ms:
            if self.getCompartment(m) == self.SUSCEPTIBLE and \
→rng.random() <= self._pRewire:
                # selected a susceptible neighbour to rewire,
                # remove its link to us
                self.removeEdge(n, m)

                # rewire to another random susceptible
                mprime = self.locus(self.SUSCEPTIBLE).draw()
                self.addEdge(m, mprime)


    def infect(self, t, e):
        (n, _) = e

        # perform a normal infection event
        super(AdaptiveSIR, self).infect(t, e)

        # quarantine the newly-infected node
        self.quarantine(n)
```

This is quite a subtle operation, so we should test that we have it coded correctly. A simple "unit test" we can perform is to check the progress of the same epidemic in two different cases for which we know what the answer should be:

- when the probability that a susceptible neighbour will be rewired, $p_{rewire} = 0$, so that no rewiring occurs (which should behave identically to normal SIR); and

- when $p_{rewire} = 1$ and all susceptible neighbours are immediately rewired, which should extinguish the epidemic with almost no infection beyond the initial "seeds".

(To expand the second point slightly, we will see the initially infected nodes infect some of their neighbours before they are removed. But those secondary infections wil be immediately and perfectly quarantined and so will have no opportunity to infect any other nodes. We'll therefore see one "generation" of secondary infections, and no more.)

We'll run the same disease for these two scenarios.

```
# network parameters
N = 2000
kmean = 40

# simulation time
T = 5000

# disease parameters
pInfected = 0.01
pInfect = 0.0001
pRemove = 0.001
```

```
# experimental parameters common to both experiments
params = dict()
params[ERNetworkDynamics.N] = N
params[ERNetworkDynamics.KMEAN] = kmean
params[epydemic.SIR.P_INFECTED] = pInfected
params[epydemic.SIR.P_INFECT] = pInfect
params[epydemic.SIR.P_REMOVE] = pRemove
params[epydemic.Monitor.DELTA] = T / 50

# create model and experiment over ER network
m = AdaptiveSIR()
```

(continues on next page)

(continued from previous page)

```
m.setMaximumTime(T)
e = ERNetworkDynamics(m)

# no rewiring
params[AdaptiveSIR.P_REWIRE] = 0.0
rc_0 = e.set(params).run()

# perfect rewiring
params[AdaptiveSIR.P_REWIRE] = 1.0
rc_1 = e.set(params).run()
```

```
(fig, axs) = plt.subplots(1, 2, sharey=True,
                          figsize=(12, 6))

# plot the two cases side by side
for (ax, rc, caption) in [ (axs[0], rc_0, 'No rewiring ($p_
→{rewire} = 0.0$)'),
                          (axs[1], rc_1, 'Perfect rewiring (
→$p_{rewire} = 1.0$)') ]:
    results = rc[epyc.Experiment.RESULTS]
    timeseries = results[epidemic.Monitor.TIMESERIES]
    ts = timeseries[epidemic.Monitor.OBSERVATIONS]
    sss = timeseries[epidemic.SIR.SUSCEPTIBLE]
    iss = timeseries[epidemic.SIR.INFECTED]
    rss = timeseries[epidemic.SIR.REMOVED]
    ax.plot(ts, sss, 'r.', label='suceptible')
    ax.plot(ts, iss, 'g.', label='infected')
    #ax.plot(ts, rss, 'ks', label='removed')
    ax.set_xlim([0, T])
    ax.set_xlabel('$t$')
    ax.set_ylim([0, N])
    ax.legend(loc='center right')
    ax.set_title(caption)

# fine-tune figure
axs[0].set_ylabel('population that is...')
fig.suptitle('SIR on ER for different rewirings ($N = {n}$, \\
→langle k \\rangle = {k}$)'.format(n=N, k=kmean), y=1.05)

_ = plt.show()
```

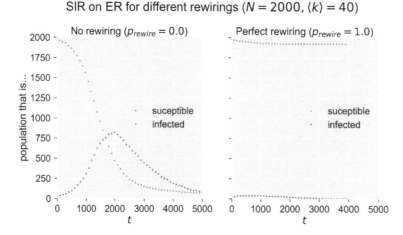

Compare the left-hand plot with those we created earlier. The right-hand plot clearly shows very minimal infection.

Having acquired some confidence in the correctness of the code, we can explore the effect of different values of p_{rewire} on the size of epidemic. We'll do this by performing experiments across the parameter range, with 100 repetitions of each to see what the variance is like.

```
lab = epyc.ClusterLab(profile='hogun', notebook=epyc.
    JSONLabNotebook('datasets/sir-quarantine.json', create=True))
```

```
lab[ERNetworkDynamics.N] = N
lab[ERNetworkDynamics.KMEAN] = kmean
lab[epydemic.SIR.P_INFECTED] = pInfected
lab[epydemic.SIR.P_INFECT] = pInfect
lab[epydemic.SIR.P_REMOVE] = pRemove
lab[epydemic.Monitor.DELTA] = T / 50

# adaptation
lab[AdaptiveSIR.P_REWIRE] = numpy.linspace(0.0, 1.0,
                                           num=100)
```

```
rc = lab.runExperiment(epyc.RepeatedExperiment(
                       epyc.RepeatedExperiment(e, 10),
                       10))
```

Asymptomatic transmission

Again this requires quite a lot of computation, but then we can plot the results.

```
df = epyc.JSONLabNotebook('datasets/sir-quarantine.json').
  ↪dataframe()
```

```
fig = plt.figure(figsize=(8, 8))
ax = fig.gca()

# plot the size of the removed population
ax.plot(df[AdaptiveSIR.P_REWIRE],
        df[epydemic.SIR.REMOVED], 'r.')
ax.set_xlabel('$p_{rewire}$')
ax.set_ylabel('population that is...')
ax.set_title('SIR epidemic size vs $p_{rewire}$ ' + '($N = {n}
  ↪, \\langle k \\rangle = {k}, '.format(n=N, k=kmean) + 'p_{\\
  ↪mathit{infect}} = ' + '{p}$)'.format(p=pInfect), y=1.05)

plt.savefig('sir-er-rewiring.png', dpi=300)
_ = plt.show()
```

SIR epidemic size vs p_{rewire} ($N = 2000$, $\langle k \rangle = 40$, $p_{infect} = 0.0001$)

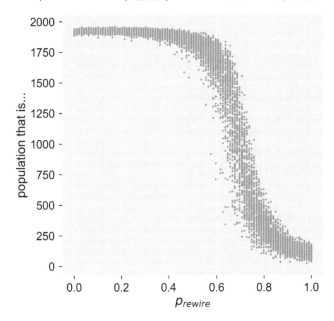

That perhaps isn't what we might have expected! At low rates of rewiring the epidemic still infects a lot of the network. But around $p_{rewire} = 0.5$ there's an abrupt change, and the size of the epidemic collapses to near zero, albeit with a lot of variance between different experiments. This suggests that there's a critical region within which rewiring (quarantine, remember) interact with detailed features of the network, so the effect is more or less dramatic depending on the exact details of how the rewiring happens.

Quarantining people before they're symptomatic

That's about all we can say about quarantine in SIR – but in SEIR we have more options. Specifically we can explore the **test, trace, and isolate** strategy by looking to quarantine people who are exposed but currently asymptomatic: in other words, when we encounter a symptomatic (infected) person, we trace their contacts, test them, and isolate any that we find to be infected.

This is the importance of SEIR as a model. It lets us explore additional countermeasures, specifically those that rely on detecting asymptomatic individuals.

Of course no such programme will be 100% effective, so alongside our probability p_{rewire} of rewiring susceptible neighbours away from infected (and now also exposed) nodes, we'll have a probability p_{detect} determining the probability that an exposed neighbour of an infected individual will be detected by the test and trace process. To be clear: p_{rewire} says how effective quarantine is, while p_{detect} says how effective testing is.

(You'll notice we just introduced two new degrees of freedom into our SEIR model: that's six parameters now, a lot to be working with.)

Again, we can add our scheme to the standard SEIR model. We'll use the same quarantine function since that process hasn't changed, but we now perform it when an exposed

node develops symptoms, and quarantine some fraction of its
neighbouring exposed nodes.

```
%%pxlocal

class AdaptiveSEIR(MonitoredSEIR):

    P_DETECT = 'pDetect'   #: Parameter for the probability
                           # of detecting an exposed
                           # neighbour of an infected node.
    P_REWIRE = 'pRewire'   #: Parameter for the probability
                           # of rewiring an SE or SI edge.

    def __init__(self):
        super(AdaptiveSEIR, self).__init__()

    def build(self, params):
        super(AdaptiveSEIR, self).build(params)

        # store the parameters for later
        self._pDetect = params[self.P_DETECT]
        self._pRewire = params[self.P_REWIRE]

    def quarantine(self, n):
        g = self.network()
        rng = numpy.random.default_rng()
        ms = list(g.neighbors(n))
        for m in ms:
            if self.getCompartment(m) == self.SUSCEPTIBLE and_
 ↪rng.random() <= self._pRewire:
                # a susceptible neighbour, remove link to us
                self.removeEdge(n, m)

                # rewire to another random susceptible
                mprime = self.locus(self.SUSCEPTIBLE).draw()
                self.addEdge(m, mprime)

    def symptoms(self, t, n):
        # perform a normal becoming-symptomatic event
        super(AdaptiveSEIR, self).symptoms(t, n)

        g = self.network()
        rng = numpy.random.default_rng()
```

(continues on next page)

(continued from previous page)

```
        # examine all neighbours and look for exposed
        # nodes to quarantine
        ms = list(g.neighbors(n))
        for m in ms:
            if self.getCompartment(m) == self.EXPOSED and rng.
↪random() <= self._pDetect:
                # detected an exposed individual,
                # quarantine them
                self.quarantine(m)

        # quarantine the newly symptomatic node
        self.quarantine(n)
```

Notice that we've got two places where we look at the neighbours of a node and decided what to do with them. In symptoms() we look for exposed neighbours, detect them with probability p_{detect}, and quarantine them if we do; in quarantine() we look for susceptible neighbours and rewire them with probability p_{rewire}. If we set $p_{detect} = 1$, our test-and-trace regime is perfect; if we set $p_{rewire} = 1$, then our isolation regime is perfect.

Again, let's unit-test the code by looking at two extreme cases, where $p_{detect} = 0$ and $p_{detect} = 1$, keeping the value of p_{rewire} the same.

```
# network parameters
N = 10000
kmean = 40

# SEIR disease parameters
pExposed = 0.001
pSymptoms = 0.002
pRemove = 0.002
pInfect = 0.000075

# adaptation
pRewire = 0.5
```

```
# experimental parameters common to both experiments
params = dict()
params[ERNetworkDynamics.N] = N
params[ERNetworkDynamics.KMEAN] = kmean
params[epydemic.SEIR.P_EXPOSED] = pExposed
params[epydemic.SEIR.P_SYMPTOMS] = pSymptoms
params[epydemic.SEIR.P_REMOVE] = pRemove
params[epydemic.SEIR.P_INFECT_SYMPTOMATIC] = pInfect
params[epydemic.SEIR.P_INFECT_ASYMPTOMATIC] = pInfect
params[epydemic.Monitor.DELTA] = T / 50
params[AdaptiveSEIR.P_REWIRE] = pRewire

# create model and experiment over ER network
m = AdaptiveSEIR()
m.setMaximumTime(T)
e = ERNetworkDynamics(m)

# no detection
params[AdaptiveSEIR.P_DETECT] = 0.0
rc_0 = e.set(params).run()

# perfect detection
params[AdaptiveSEIR.P_DETECT] = 1.0
rc_1 = e.set(params).run()
```

```
(fig, axs) = plt.subplots(1, 2, sharey=True, figsize=(12, 6))

# plot the two cases side by side
for (ax, rc, caption) in [ (axs[0], rc_0, 'No detection ($p_
↪{detect} = 0.0$)'),
                           (axs[1], rc_1, 'Perfect detection (
↪$p_{detect} = 1.0$)') ]:
    results = rc[epyc.Experiment.RESULTS]
    timeseries = results[epydemic.Monitor.TIMESERIES]
    ts = timeseries[epydemic.Monitor.OBSERVATIONS]
    sss = timeseries[epydemic.SEIR.SUSCEPTIBLE]
    ess = timeseries[epydemic.SEIR.EXPOSED]
    iss = timeseries[epydemic.SEIR.INFECTED]
    rss = timeseries[epydemic.SEIR.REMOVED]
    ax.plot(ts, sss, 'r.', label='suceptible')
    ax.plot(ts, ess, 'b.', label='exposed')
    ax.plot(ts, iss, 'g.', label='infected')
```

(continues on next page)

Quarantining people before they're symptomatic   **147**

(continued from previous page)

```
#ax.plot(ts, rss, 'ks', label='removed')
ax.set_xlim([0, T])
ax.set_xlabel('$t$')
ax.set_ylim([0, N])
ax.legend(loc='center left')
ax.set_title(caption)

# fine-tune figure
axs[0].set_ylabel('population that is...')
fig.suptitle('SEIR on ER for different detection of exposed␣
 ↪individuals ($N = {n}, \\langle k \\rangle = {k}'.format(n=N,
 ↪ k=kmean) + ', p_{rewire} = ' + '{p}$)'.format(p=pRewire),␣
 ↪y=1.05)

_ = plt.show()
```

SEIR on ER for different detection of exposed individuals ($N = 10000, \langle k \rangle = 40, p_{rewire} = 0.5$)

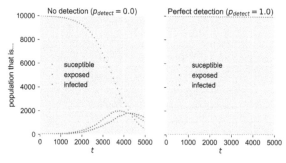

With no detection (in the left-hand plot) of exposed nodes we see an epidemic break out, albeit quite a small one. The exposed nodes start spreading infection silently, but since they're never detected the only countermeasures that happen are a 50%-effective quarantine of infected nodes. In the right-hand plot the perfect detection means that the countermeasures are very effective, even when the quarantine is only 50% effective.

Let's see what effect detection efficiency has. Remember, p_{detect} is the probability that an exposed neighbour of an infected individual will be detected and then quarantined: you can think of it as a measure of how effectively we're doing the "test" and "trace" parts of "test, trace, and isolate". We probably expect that a more effective detection regime – where more exposed individuals are detected earlier – will have the effect of reducing the size of the epidemic.

```
lab = epyc.ClusterLab(profile='hogun', notebook=epyc.
  JSONLabNotebook('datasets/seir-quarantine.json',
  create=True))
```

We need to pick values for the other parameters in the model, so let's rather arbitrarily say that asymptomatic and symptomatic infection happen with the same probability, and that we have a quarantine regime that's 50%-effective both for infected people and for those we uncover through testing.

```
lab[ERNetworkDynamics.N] = N
lab[ERNetworkDynamics.KMEAN] = kmean

lab[epydemic.SEIR.P_EXPOSED] = 0.001
lab[epydemic.SEIR.P_REMOVE] = 0.002
lab[epydemic.SEIR.P_INFECT_ASYMPTOMATIC] = 0.000075
lab[epydemic.SEIR.P_INFECT_SYMPTOMATIC] = 0.000075
lab[epydemic.SEIR.P_SYMPTOMS] = 0.002
lab[epydemic.Monitor.DELTA] = T / 50

# adaptation
pRewire = 0.5
lab[AdaptiveSEIR.P_REWIRE] = pRewire
lab[AdaptiveSEIR.P_DETECT] = numpy.linspace(0.0, 1.0,
                                            num=100)
```

```
m = AdaptiveSEIR()
e = ERNetworkDynamics(m)
rc = lab.runExperiment(epyc.RepeatedExperiment(
                    epyc.RepeatedExperiment(e, 10),
                10))
```

More simulation results in the following.

```
df = epyc.JSONLabNotebook('datasets/seir-quarantine.json').
  dataframe()
```

```
fig = plt.figure(figsize=(8, 8))
ax = fig.gca()

# plot the size of the removed population
results = df[df[AdaptiveSEIR.P_REWIRE] == pRewire]
ax.plot(results[AdaptiveSEIR.P_DETECT],
        results[epydemic.SEIR.REMOVED], 'r.')
ax.set_xlabel('$p_{detect}$')
ax.set_ylabel('population that is...')
ax.set_title('SEIR epidemic size vs $p_{detect}}$ ' + '($N =
→{n}, \\langle k \\rangle = {k}, '.format(n=N, k=kmean) + 'p_
→{rewire} = ' + '{p}$)'.format(p=pRewire), y=1.05)

_ = plt.show()
```

SEIR epidemic size vs p_{detect} ($N = 10000$, $\langle k \rangle = 40$, $p_{rewire} = 0.5$)

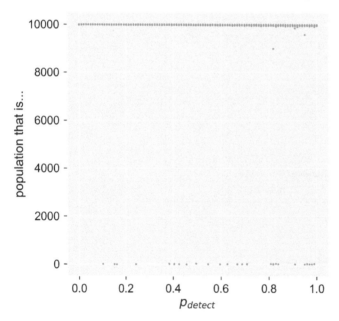

Perhaps a little disappointing: it seems that detection doesn't
have much effect in this case. You'll notice that it's not *no* effect:
there are cases right across the graph in which the size of the
outbreak is around zero, but in the majority of cases there is a
large epidemic.

Might this be to do with the effectiveness of quarantine? If we adopt an 80%-effective regime, what then happens?

```
pRewire = 0.8
```

```
lab[AdaptiveSEIR.P_REWIRE] = pRewire
rc = lab.runExperiment(epyc.RepeatedExperiment(
                        epyc.RepeatedExperiment(e, 10),
                  10))
```

```
df = epyc.JSONLabNotebook('datasets/seir-quarantine.json').
 ⌐dataframe()
```

```
fig = plt.figure(figsize=(8, 8))
ax = fig.gca()

# plot the size of the removed population
results = df[df[AdaptiveSEIR.P_REWIRE] == pRewire]
ax.plot(results[AdaptiveSEIR.P_DETECT],
        results[epydemic.SEIR.REMOVED], 'r.')
ax.set_xlabel('$p_{detect}$')
ax.set_ylabel('population that is...')
ax.set_title('SEIR epidemic size vs $p_{detect}}$ ' + '($N =
 ⌐{n}, \\langle k \\rangle = {k}, '.format(n=N, k=kmean) + 'p_
 ⌐{rewire} = ' + '{p}$)'.format(p=pRewire), y=1.05)

plt.savefig('seir-er-rewiring.png', dpi=300)
_ = plt.show()
```

SEIR epidemic size vs p_{detect} ($N = 10000$, $\langle k \rangle = 40$, $p_{rewire} = 0.5$)

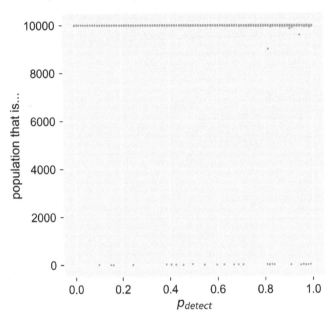

Very different! What are we seeing?

Firstly, notice that in almost all cases we have some examples of epidemics with very small outbreaks, suggesting that even low detection rates *can* make a difference. But at low values of p_{detect} that difference is really rather sparse: it doesn't happen often.

As p_{detect} increases – that is, as testing and tracing becomes more effective, we start to see a strange effect: a "waterfall" of results. Remember that each point on the graph represents a single experimental epidemic. Within the waterfall, some of these experiments have huge outbreaks, some have none, and some fall in between. This may suggest that the really detailed structure of the network makes a difference: some small thing is enough to change the way the stochastic process evolves and so swing the results.

Then as we continue to increase p_{detect} we see something else. The "waterfall" continues, but suddenly there are no really large outbreaks. Detection and quarantine aren't stopping epidemics from happening, but they *are* limiting their size. Finally we see very effective control when we have perfect detection – although still *imperfect* control, because of the imperfect quarantine.

Questions for discussion

- What sort of detection activities might you impose in an epidemic? How effective would it be? What could you do to make it *more* effective?

- What would happen if you had vaccination *and* test, trace, and isolate in place at the same time? Would one compensate for weaknesses in the other?

Physical distancing

Quarantine seems to be very effective, especially when carried out strongly enough and when combined with effective detection of exposed individuals. But you need to get a lot right for it to work. Maybe there's another way?

Let's go back to basics. In SEIR-style diseases we have the possibility of individuals walking around and spreading the disease without showing any symptoms. There is by definition no way (absent testing) to spot these individuals until (and unless) they show symptoms. So the challenge is to stop these infectious-but-asymptomatic individuals from coming into contact with susceptible individuals.

What if we re-structure the contact network so that people only have contact with a small group of people, and reduce the amount of mixing between those groups? If someone is infected in spite of everything then they'll probably infect their own group, but they'll be less opportunity to infect other groups. This strategy is referred to as **physical distancing**, reducing and re-structuring the connections within a population.

Some people *never* develop symptoms: for some reason their immune systems suppress the disease enough to keep them well, but not enough to eliminate it and stop them being infectious. The most famous case of this phenomenon is "Typhoid Mary" , who infected a large number of people with typhoid fever despite showing no symptoms herself.

Filio Marinelli, Gregory Tsoucalas, Marianna Karaminou, and George Androutsos. Mary Mallon (1869–1938) and the history of typhoid fever. *Annals of Gastroenterology*, 26(2):123–134, 2013

A physically-distanced contact network

Physical distancing is another topological approach to epidemic control. It works by changing the network over which the disease operates, rather than addressing the disease itself. Such approach is well-suited to new diseases and those for which there are few effective therapies.

What does "physical distancing" mean in network terms? We can understand it best by thinking about the actual conditions of socially-distant lockdown, and then re-creating this structure as a network.

The idea of physical distancing is to place individuals in small "bubbles" of contact – typically just their own immediate family – with whom they interact strongly, and weaken the connections that any family member has with individuals in other bubbles. Within a bubble, infection of one person will probably transfer quickly to most or all all of the other members. But the ability of the disease to pass between bubbles is substantially reduced, since there is relatively little contact between them. One can reduce the inter-bubble transmission even further using quarantine when someone realises they are infected.

Sometimes referred to as **social distancing**, although that feels like an oxymoron: it also sounds uncomfortably close to "social isolation", which indeed is one of its major dangers as a technique.

In network terms, the bubbles are complete graphs (everyone in a bubble meets everyone else) whose size depends on the size of the family. We could set all families to the same size, say 4; alternatively we could draw family sizes from some probability distribution where the average size of a family is 4.5 (2 adults with the proverbial 2.5 children) but we allow larger and smaller families to occur. Larger families risk more infections if a member is infected.

We now need to link the bubbles. In each bubble, some person or people meet with the outside world: perhaps they're the designated shopper, or someone in a key role whose work brings them into contact with others. We then need to connect these people to other bubbles.

This description still leaves quite a lot to be decided:

- What is the distribution of family sizes? Are large families really unusual? Or do they follow a "normal" distribution?

- How many people in each family connect to the outside? Is it always one or two? Might a large family have more contacts?

- How do those in contact outside their family group connect with others? Are some people significantly more connected than others?

These decisions are simply additional degrees of freedom (again) for our model – with all that this entails.

Creating such a network means addressing all these issues. There's a trick we can perform, though. Notice that while the detailed choices change, the structure of the network doesn't. This means that, just as our disease models have parameters that we can change, so does our socially-distanced network – with the difference that the network parameters are given by choices of probability distributions as well as single numbers. But the solution is the same: define what it means to build the network, providing these distributions as parameters that are "plugged in" to the same structure-building process.

Building the network involves a complicated piece of code – the most complicated we've seen so far.

```
def distanced_graph(N, clusterSizeDistribution,
    contactDistribution, clusterContactDistribution):
    # build the initial graph
    g = networkx.Graph()

    # build the clusters, each being a complete
    # graph K_s of size s, labelled uniquely
    # within the overall graph
    rng = numpy.random.default_rng()
    n = 0
    cid = 1
    clusters = []
    while n < N:
        # build the cluster's graph with a random size
        s = clusterSizeDistribution()
        K_s = networkx.complete_graph(s)

        # relabel the cluster graph so all nodes in the final
        # social distence graph have unique integer labels
        networkx.relabel_nodes(K_s, lambda l: n + l,
                               copy=False)
```

(continues on next page)

(continued from previous page)

```
    # add to the graph and list of clusters
    # label edges with the cluster they belong to
    # (numbered from 1) and the size of the cluster
    g.add_nodes_from(K_s.nodes,
                     cluster=cid, cluster_size=s)
    g.add_edges_from(K_s.edges,
                     cluster=cid, cluster_size=s)
    clusters.append(K_s)
    n += s
    cid += 1

# draw the number of contact nodes per cluster from
# from the distribution
contacts = []
for c in clusters:
    s = c.order()
    d = contactDistribution(s)
    contacts.append(d)

# decide on the arity of each contact node
stubs = []
for i in range(len(clusters)):
    c = clusters[i]
    # first i node labels (since all nodes are
    # identical in K_s)
    ls = list(c.nodes())[:contacts[i]]
    for l in ls:
        # draw the number of contacts for this node
        e = clusterContactDistribution(n)

        # append e copies of the node label to
        # the list of stubs
        stubs.extend([l] * e)

# if number of stubs isn't even, add one to a
# randomly-chosen node (don't favour
# already-high-degree nodes
if len(stubs) % 2 > 0:
    us = list(set(stubs))
    j = rng.integers(len(us))
    stubs.append(us[j])
```

(continues on next page)

(continued from previous page)

```
# shuffle the stubs until there are no edge
# pair with the same endpoints
rng.shuffle(stubs)  # may leave loops
while True:
    # look for pairtings of stubs and others
    # within the same cluster, and break them
    # randomly (without changing the degree
    # distribution)
    swaps = 0
    for i in range(0, len(stubs), 2):
        if g.nodes[stubs[i]]['cluster'] == g.nodes[stubs[i
↪+ 1]]['cluster']:
            # self loop, swap with another
            # randomly-chosen stub
            j = rng.integers(len(stubs))
            t = stubs[i + 1]
            stubs[i + 1] = stubs[j]
            stubs[j] = t

            swaps += 1
    if swaps == 0:
        # no swaps, we're finished
        break

# connect the nodes by pulling pairs of stubs
# and creating an edge between them
for i in range(0, len(stubs), 2):
    # label inter-bubble edges as cluster 0 of size 0
    g.add_edge(stubs[i], stubs[i + 1],
               cluster=0, cluster_size=0)

# return the graph and list of cluster sizes
return (g, list(map(lambda h: h.order(), clusters)))
```

This function takes four parameters – the size of network and three probability-distribution functions – and returns a network and a list of the bubble sizes. Within the network it creates the social bubbles and labels them uniquely, and then connects the bubbles together randomly.

A physically-distanced contact network

Making some choices

We can't get away from making choices about these degrees of
freedom indefinitely, though – and in fact that time has arrived.

Since we're interested in large-scale phenomena, let's make some
simple choices:

- Families whose sizes are normally-distributed integers with a
  mean of 4.5 and a standard deviation of 2

- A normal distribution of contacts in each family

- Exponentially-distributed links betyween connections, to
  allow for very connected individuals

Since it makes no sense to allow entirely isolated families, those
with no size, and "connected" individuals with no contacts, we
cut off all the distributions with a minimum of 1.

```
def averageFamily():
    rng = numpy.random.default_rng()
    return max(int(rng.normal(4.5, 2)), 1)
```

```
def coupleOfContacts(s):
    rng = numpy.random.default_rng()
    return max(int(rng.normal(min(s / 2, 2), 1)), 1)
```

```
def expInterBubble(n):
    rng = numpy.random.default_rng()
    return max(int(rng.exponential(10.0)), 1)
```

These three functions, coupled with the network size, are enough
to build our network.

```
N = 1000
```

```
(g, clusters) = distanced_graph(N, averageFamily,␣
␣coupleOfContacts, expInterBubble)
```

We can check the various elements of this network. For example, we can check what range of family "bubble" sizes we have, and how connected the various contact individuals are.

```
print('Mean family size of {s:.2f} (range {minf}-{maxf})'.
 ↪format(s=numpy.mean(clusters), minf=min(clusters),␣
 ↪maxf=max(clusters)))
print('Most connected individual has {k} contacts'.
 ↪format(k=max(dict(g.degree()).values())))
```

```
Mean family size of 4.00 (range 1-10)
Most connected individual has 55 contacts
```

We could also draw the network to inspect it, colouring the nodes with the size of cluster they belong to – although that turns out not to be especially revealing.

```
def draw_distanced(g, cmap=None,
                    color='cluster_size',
                    ax=None):
    # fill in defaults
    if cmap is None:
        cmap = plt.get_cmap('viridis')
    if ax is None:
        ax = plt.gca()

    # work out the colours
    ncs = list(map(lambda n: g.nodes[n][color],
                g.nodes()))
    ecs = list(map(lambda e: g.edges[e][color],
                g.edges()))

    # draw with spring layout, which seems to
    # give good results
    networkx.draw_spring(g,
                    ax=ax,
                    with_labels=False,
                    node_size=50,
                    node_color=ncs,
                    edge_color=ecs,
                    cmap=cmap,
                    edge_cmap=cmap)
```

(continues on next page)

(continued from previous page)

```python
fig = plt.figure(figsize=(12, 12))
ax = fig.gca()

# draw network
cmap = plt.get_cmap('viridis')
draw_distanced(g, cmap=cmap)

# add key (see https://matplotlib.org/examples/api/colorbar_
 →only.html)
bounds = list(range(min(clusters), max(clusters)))
norm = matplotlib.colors.BoundaryNorm(bounds, cmap.N)
ax1 = fig.add_axes([0.95, 0.15, 0.05, 0.7])
cb2 = matplotlib.colorbar.ColorbarBase(ax1, cmap=cmap,
                                norm=norm,
                                boundaries=bounds,
                                ticks=bounds,
                                spacing='proportional',
                                orientation='vertical')

plt.savefig('physical-distancing.png', dpi=300)
_ = plt.show()
```

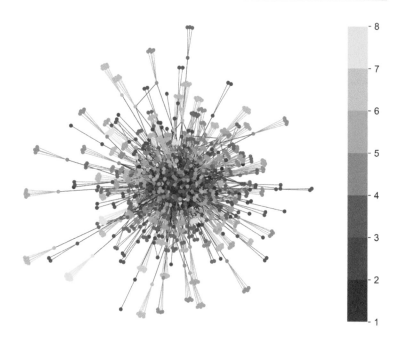

This isn't a useless plot, once we know that more highly-connected clusters sit in the centre with less-connected clusters pushed to the outside. We can see these less-connected clusters, and in particular see that they have a range of colours, indicating that they're of different sizes – and therefore giving confidence that the algorithm hasn't (for example) only made large clusters highly connected.

Disease and distancing

Now we can run a disease process over our network. We'll stick to SIR to reduce the number of degrees of freedom we have to deal with: running with SEIR would be easy to do too, of course, but presents us with even more choices.

What do we expect from a disease in these circumstances? The purpose of physical distancing is to reduce the connectivity of people, which (all things being equal) should reduce the disease's spread. But it does so by building tight clusters of individuals within bubbles, meaning that infecting one person is likely to infect everyone. And we've used an exponential distribution of contacts to allow the creation of high-degree hubs, meaning that infecting one of these will potentially infect a lot of others.

The best we can probably say at this stage, then, is that ... it's complicated. Which is just the sort of situation simulation is intended for.

```
lab = epyc.ClusterLab(profile='hogun',
                    notebook=epyc.JSONLabNotebook('datasets/
 ↪sir-phydist.json', create=True))
```

If we cast the above code into a format suitable for running as an experiment, we can then look at how an epidemic proceeds for a sample point in the parameter space.

```
%%pxlocal

class PhyDistNetworkDynamics(epydemic.StochasticDynamics):

    # Experimental parameters
    N = 'N'
    BUBBLE_MEAN = 'bubbleMean'
    BUBBLE_STDDEV = 'bubbleStddev'
    INTERBUBBLE_EXP= 'interBubbleExp'

    def __init__(self, p):
        super(PhyDistNetworkDynamics, self).__init__(p)

    def bubbleSize(self):
        rng = numpy.random.default_rng()
        return max(int(rng.normal(self._bubbleMean,
                                  self._bubbleStddev)), 1)

    def contacts(self, s):
        rng = numpy.random.default_rng()
        return max(int(rng.normal(min(s / 2, 2), 1)), 1)

    def interBubble(self):
        rng = numpy.random.default_rng()
        return max(int(rng.exponential(self._
→interBubbleExponent)), 1)

    def distanced(self, N):
        g = networkx.Graph()

        rng = numpy.random.default_rng()
        n = 0
        cid = 1
        clusters = []
        while n < N:
            s = self.bubbleSize()
            K_s = networkx.complete_graph(s)

            networkx.relabel_nodes(K_s,
                                   lambda l: n + l, copy=False)
            g.add_nodes_from(K_s.nodes,
                             cluster=cid, cluster_size=s)
            g.add_edges_from(K_s.edges,
```

(continues on next page)

(continued from previous page)

```
                          cluster=cid, cluster_size=s)
        clusters.append(K_s)
        n += s
        cid += 1

    contacts = []
    for c in clusters:
        s = c.order()
        d = self.contacts(s)
        contacts.append(d)

    stubs = []
    for i in range(len(clusters)):
        c = clusters[i]
        ls = list(c.nodes())[:contacts[i]]
        for l in ls:
            e = self.interBubble()
            stubs.extend([l] * e)
    if len(stubs) % 2 > 0:
        us = list(set(stubs))
        j = rng.integers(len(us))
        stubs.append(us[j])

    rng.shuffle(stubs)
    while True:
        swaps = 0
        for i in range(0, len(stubs), 2):
            if g.nodes[stubs[i]]['cluster'] == g.
→nodes[stubs[i + 1]]['cluster']:
                j = rng.integers(len(stubs))
                t = stubs[i + 1]
                stubs[i + 1] = stubs[j]
                stubs[j] = t
                swaps += 1
        if swaps == 0:
            break

    for i in range(0, len(stubs), 2):
        g.add_edge(stubs[i], stubs[i + 1],
                   cluster=0, cluster_size=0)

    return g
```

(continues on next page)

(continued from previous page)

```
    def configure(self, params):
        super(PhyDistNetworkDynamics, self).configure(params)

        N = params[self.N]
        self._bubbleMean = params[self.BUBBLE_MEAN]
        self._bubbleStddev = params[self.BUBBLE_STDDEV]
        self._interBubbleExponent = params[self.INTERBUBBLE_
EXP]

        g = self.distanced(N)
        self.setNetworkPrototype(g)
```

```
# network size
N = 10000

# simulation time
T = 5000

# disease parameters
pInfected = 0.01
pInfect = 0.0003
pRemove = 0.002
```

```
# experimental parameters common to both experiments
params = dict()
params[PhyDistNetworkDynamics.N] = 10000
params[PhyDistNetworkDynamics.BUBBLE_MEAN] = 4.5
params[PhyDistNetworkDynamics.BUBBLE_STDDEV] = 2.0
params[PhyDistNetworkDynamics.INTERBUBBLE_EXP] = 10.0
params[epydemic.SIR.P_INFECTED] = pInfected
params[epydemic.SIR.P_INFECT] = pInfect
params[epydemic.SIR.P_REMOVE] = pRemove
params[epydemic.Monitor.DELTA] = T / 50

# create model and experiment over distance network
m = MonitoredSIR()
m.setMaximumTime(T)
e = PhyDistNetworkDynamics(m)

rc = e.set(params).run()
```

```
fig = plt.figure(figsize=(8, 8))
ax = fig.gca()

timeseries = rc[epyc.Experiment.RESULTS][epidemic.Monitor.
 ↪TIMESERIES]
tss = timeseries[epydemic.Monitor.OBSERVATIONS]
sss = timeseries[epydemic.SIR.SUSCEPTIBLE]
iss = timeseries[epydemic.SIR.INFECTED]
rss = timeseries[epydemic.SIR.REMOVED]
ax.plot(tss, sss, 'r-', label='susceptible')
ax.plot(tss, iss, 'g-', label='infected')
#ax.plot(tss, rss, 'k-', label='removed')
ax.set_xlabel('$t$')
ax.set_ylabel('population that is...')
ax.legend(loc='center right')

# fine-time the figure
ax.set_title('SIR on a physically distant network ($p_{\mathit
 ↪{infect}} = ' + '{p}$)'.format(p=pInfect), y=1.05)

_ = plt.show()
```

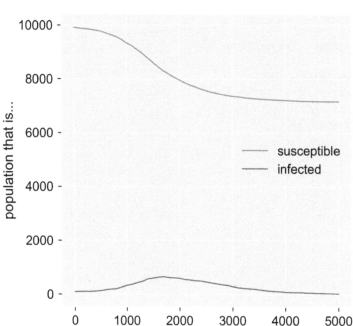

SIR on a physically distant network ($p_{infect} = 0.0003$)

Compare this to the same disease on an ER network. The epidemic doesn't really get started in the network, even for a value of p_{infect} that previous experience would suggest would be sufficient. We can explore this by checking the size of the epidemic across a range of infectiousness values.

```
# network parameters
lab[PhyDistNetworkDynamics.N] = 10000
lab[PhyDistNetworkDynamics.BUBBLE_MEAN] = 4.5
lab[PhyDistNetworkDynamics.BUBBLE_STDDEV] = 2.0
lab[PhyDistNetworkDynamics.INTERBUBBLE_EXP] = 10.0

# disease parameters
lab[epydemic.SIR.P_INFECTED] = pInfected
lab[epydemic.SIR.P_INFECT] = numpy.linspace(0.0, 0.0008,
                                            num=100)
lab[epydemic.SIR.P_REMOVE] = pRemove

lab[epydemic.Monitor.DELTA] = T / 50
```

```
m = MonitoredSIR()
m.setMaximumTime(T)
e = PhyDistNetworkDynamics(m)
lab.runExperiment(epyc.RepeatedExperiment(
                    epyc.RepeatedExperiment(e, 10),
                10))
```

```
df = epyc.JSONLabNotebook('datasets/sir-phydist.json').
  dataframe()
```

```
fig = plt.figure(figsize=(8, 8))
ax = fig.gca()

# plot the size of the removed population
ax.plot(df[epydemic.SIR.P_INFECT],
        df[epydemic.SIR.REMOVED], 'r,')
ax.set_xlabel('$p_{\\mathit{infect}}$')
ax.set_ylabel('population that is...')
ax.set_title('SIR with physical distancing ($N = {n}$)'.
  format(n=N), y=1.05)

plt.savefig('sir-phydist.png', dpi=300)
plt.show()
```

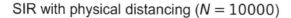

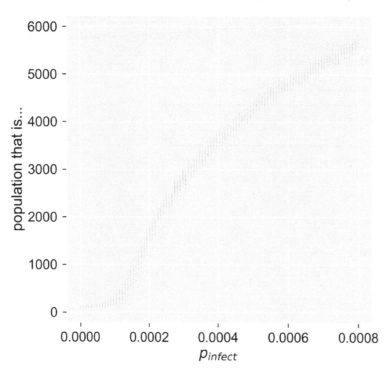

SIR with physical distancing ($N = 10000$)

Comparing this with the same disease on ER networks we see that the epidemic takes off similarly. Why is this? – it would need more exploration, but the way we set up the socially distanced model did include powerlaw-distributed contacts between bubbles. It could be that these superspreaders are responsible for spreading the disease between bubbles, at which point is spreads easily within them.

This brings up an important point about social distancing, and in particular about how to weaken such a lockdown. The size of bubbles, and their interconnection doesn't matter **as long as there is no infection present in the bubble** – but it matters critically when there *is* infection, and especially if one of the bubble's contact points is highly connected. This makes the issue of acceptable behaviour very important, since smaller, more isolated, bubbles will both incur less infection within themselves (since there are fewer people) and potentially transmit less (by having fewer outside contacts).

Questions for discussion

- The case of Typhoid Mary raises some troubling questions. Is it right to lock someone up when they're done nothing personally wrong, to protect the community? What alternatives were there, before treatments like antibiotics were available? What might we do today?

- Physical distancing doesn't have to be uniform for everyone. Some people are in more need of protection ("shielding") than others. How could we introduce this into a model?

Conclusion

Many are fleeing, everyone is fearful, you are neither – splendid, magnificent! For what is more foolish than to fear what you cannot avoid by any strategy, and what you aggravate by fearing? What is more useless than to flee what will always confront you wherever you may flee?

—Petrarch, *Letters of Old Age.*

What, then, can we conclude from this brief and superficial look at epidemic modelling on networks? I would like to think that there are several broad take-away messages.

The most important message by far is that – despite using advanced mathematics, detailed sets of {index}parameters `<parameter>`, and extensive computer {index}simulation` – modelling remains an inexact science. It's important to qualify that word "inexact": while models and simulations can generate results in extraordinary volume and with great precision, the *interpretation* of those results inevitably involves judgement calls. Many details remain unknown, and in many cases unknowable, perhaps because they cannot be properly measured, or perhaps because they change so fast that measurement is quickly outdated by events. Whatever the reason, no model *in itself* tells us anything; rather, they provide evidence to guide our thinking.

A corollary to this is that the policy responses to an epidemic can only partially be driven by, determined by, or justified by, the results of modelling. Policy remains an essentially political activity, and while it may be "driven by" or "informed by" science, there will always be other factors needing to be included that may skew a final decision away from what a scientist may view as "correct". Many real-world problems are *wicked*, impossible to solve because of inherent contradictions and the compromises they imply, but mandating an immediate response nonetheless.

In many ways this makes modelling *more* important, not less. A model provides only a limited view onto any problem. But the fact that it can provide a view onto *any* problem means that we can explore problems we haven't yet faced, explore techniques we couldn't yet deploy in reality, and so forth. It is at least important to understand things that *can't* happen as it is to understand those that *can*, if only to cut down the space of possibilities that need further consideration.

The second take-away message is the scientific underpinnings of many policies with which we're familiar – so much so that they sometimes feel almost part of the world's folklore. Vaccination, quarantine, physical distancing, herd immunity, and so forth are all susceptible to exploration and variation. And the science can expose commonalities that are not initially obvious: that the provision of protective equipment behaves like vaccination, for example, in the way it can be used to reduce the dangers of super-spreading. This can lead to alternative approaches.

The third message concerns countermeasures. We saw when we discussed adaptive countermeasures that variations in the efficacy with which the processes were carried out made a huge difference to the results. In the real world, of course, one may be *stuck* with ineffective processes: an imprecise test, a limited number of testers-and-tracers, and so forth. This may defeat even a well-thought-through strategy.

The implication of this is that to impose any set of countermeasures is to **conduct an experiment** – and the same is true of any attempt to unwind a countermeasure, such as for example when coming our of a physical distancing lockdown. It's possible that the strategy will fail, and that measures will need to be re-imposed. This may be difficult for people to take, especially if they've not been warned of the possibility beforehand.

The final message is the most important for me as an academic: the *democracy* of science. People sometimes feel that science is something alien, requiring endless qualifications, state or corporate sponsorship, and access to techniques and tools that are out of reach of the amateur. Nothing could be further from the truth.

Science, as practiced by real scientists, is largely just an exerciseb *scientific method* – that has evolved over the years to help stop us misleading ourselves. The framework isn't a barrier to entry into science; rather, it's a guide to help identify simple truth within a complex reality.

The quotation from Rovelli with which we opened this book highlights that the conclusions drawn by science are always tentative and open to question, refutation, and overthrow. It's working within this framework that makes a practice into science, not the letters after the practitioner's name. And while we hope that well-qualified people are right sufficiently often to be trusted, that's an authority that has to be earned and justified by a willingness to accept correction as part of the process of truth-finding.

If this book shows anything, I hope it's that computational science is within the reach of everyone. It's not the preserve of academics, although academic scientists have developed many of the ideas and tools; it doesn't need supercomputers, although they're often useful; and no-one should be afraid of posing questions: any question, sincerely asked, is worth asking, and worth the cost of working towards an answer.

To find out more

To learn more about historical epidemics

The 1918 or "Spanish" flu is very much in the news close to its centenary. Spinney's book is the definitive source [21].

The Black Death of the fourteenth century has had a huge number of histories written about it – and to show that history is a process and not a state, is still generating new works that encourage us to revisit both the sociology and the science. Ziegler addresses the full sweep [22]; Hatcher explores it from the perspective of a village [23]; while Sloane deals with a capital city [24]. The plague also had a unique and extensive effect on literature, being observed by many writers including the poet Petrarch, who wrote extensively of its effects on Florence [25]. An accessible yet detailed scientific treatment is still waiting to be written.

To learn about epidemiology in practice

The European Centre for Disease Prevention and Control's field epidemiology manual [26] is an open-source collaboration intended as a field guide and training resource for epidemiologists in the midst of an epidemic. A dose of reality on top of theoretical treatments.

[21] Laura Spinney. *Pale Rider: The Spanish flu epidemic of 1918 and how it changed the world.* Vintage, 2018

[22] Philip Ziegler. *The Black Death.* Sutton, 2003

[23] John Hatcher. *The Black Death: An intimate story of a village in crisis, 1345–1350.* Phoenix, 2009

[24] Barney Sloane. *The Black Death in London.* The History Press, 2011

[25] Paula Findlen. Petrarch's plague: Love, death, and friendship in a time of pandemic. *The Public Domain Review,* June 2020

[26] Various authors. *Field epidemiology manual wiki.* European Centre for Disease Prevention and Control, 2019

To learn more about network science

As well as being one of the scientific pioneers, Albert-Lászl'o Barabási has written extensively and accessibly about complex networks and their applications. His book *Linked: the new science of networks* [27] is probably the best-known introductory work, with the follow-up on "bursty" processes [28] also well worth reading.

For a more social science perspective, Watts' book on small worlds [29] explores issue such as rumour spreading and the ways in which different social structures can be understood mathematically.

Textbooks and reference works on network science

The absolute best textbook on the mathematics of networks is that by Newman, another pioneer of the field [30]. Sayama deals with networks as part of a wider introduction to modelling complex systems [31]. Porter and Gleeson have produced a freely-available tutorial [32]. Kiss, Miller, and Simon's book on epidemic spreading on networks is probably the most comprehensive recent mathematical treatment, and has some associated Python code [33].

To do your own experiments

All the simulations done in this book use code that's either contained in the book itself or available in public-domain libraries. All code, diagrams, and generated datasets for this book are available for download from the project's GitHub repo, where you will also find the `requirements.txt` file needed to create a Python virtual environment capable of running everything (or indeed of re-creating the book in its entirety).

There's nothing exclusive about science, so please feel free to

[27] Albert-László Barabási. *Linked: The new science of networks.* Perseus, 2003

[28] Albert-László Barabási. *Bursts: The hidden patterns behind everything you do, from your e-mail to the Bloody Crusades.* Plume, 2011

[29] Duncan Watts. *Small worlds.* Princeton Studies in Complexity. Princeton University Press, 1999

[30] M.E.J. Newman. *Networks: an introduction.* Oxford University Press, 2010

[31] Hiroki Sayama. *Introduction to the modeling and analysis of complex systems.* SUNY Open Textbooks, 2015

[32] Mason Porter and James Gleeson. Dynamical systems on networks: a tutorial. Technical Report arXiv:1403.7663v1, arXiv, 2014

[33] István Kiss, Joel Miller, and Péter Simon. *Mathematics of epidemics on networks*, volume 46 of *Interdisciplinary Applied Mathematics.* Springer-Verlag, 2017

download the code and run your own experiments – and then please share them, and your results, with the community! You're then essentially engaging in the same processes of modelling, simulation, and experimentation as professional researchers.

Notes on production

Writing this book has meant bringing together text, mathematics, and code, using a large array of open-source tools. It's amazing what you can get your hands on these days, and I'm grateful to the contributors to the various projects for their creativity and generosity.

The book is written with a combination of "markdown" text and Jupyter notebooks to allow executable content. It was then assembled using Jupyter Book to drive the Sphinx documentation generator, and hosted on GitHub Pages.

The book is typeset by letting Sphinx drive the LaTeX typesetting system. The style is based on Edward Tufte's books on scientific visualisation, as implemented by the Tufte-LaTeX Developers.

Simulations are all written in Python 3 and expressed using the `epidemic` library for network simulation, which itself is built on top of the `networkx` library for representing and manipulating networks in Python.

The mathematics makes heavy use of the `numpy`. The diagrams are all generated using `matplotlib` together with `seaborn` to improve the graphical presentation, as well as some of the network visualisation functions built into `networkx`.

For the experiments where a lot of numbers are being crunched we use the `epyc` computational experiment management library and `pandas` to handle the resulting datasets. The large experiments use a compute cluster ("hogun") with 11 machines each with 16Gb of memory and two 4-core Intel Xeon E3-1240@3.4MHz processors; all other experiments are performed on a 2017-vintage MacBook Pro with 16Gb of memory and a dual-core Intel i5@3.1GHz processor.

All text, code, and diagrams are available for download from the project's GitHub repo.

Bibliography

[1] Réka Albert and Albert-László Barabási. Statistical mechanics of complex networks. *Reviews of Modern Physics*, 74:47–97, January 2002.

[2] Christian Althous. Estimating the reproduction number of Zaire ebolavirus (EBOV) during the 2014 outbreak in West Africa. *PLOS Currents Outbreaks*, September 2014.

[3] Various authors. *Field epidemiology manual wiki*. European Centre for Disease Prevention and Control, 2019.

[4] Albert-László Barabási. *Linked: The new science of networks*. Perseus, 2003.

[5] Albert-László Barabási. *Bursts: The hidden patterns behind everything you do, from your e-mail to the Bloody Crusades*. Plume, 2011.

[6] Paul Erdős and Alfred Renyi. On random graphs. *Publicationes Mathematicæ*, 6:290–297, 1959.

[7] Paula Findlen. Petrarch's plague: Love, death, and friendship in a time of pandemic. *The Public Domain Review*, June 2020.

[8] John Hatcher. *The Black Death: An intimate story of a village in crisis, 1345–1350*. Phoenix, 2009.

[9] Herbert Hethcote. The mathematics of infectious diseases. *SIAM Review*, 42(4):599–653, December 2000.

[10] Paul Hoffman. *The man who loved only numbers: The story of Paul Erdős and the search for mathematical truth*. Hyperion, 1998.

[11] Jeffrey Kephart and Steve White. Directed-graph epidemiological models of computer viruses. In *Proceedings of Research in Security and Privacy*, pages 343–359. IEEE Press, May 1991.

[12] István Kiss, Joel Miller, and Péter Simon. *Mathematics of epidemics on networks*, volume 46 of *Interdisciplinary Applied Mathematics*. Springer-Verlag, 2017.

[13] Peter Mann, John Mitchell, V. Anne Smith, and Simon Dobson. Percolation in random graphs with higher-order clustering. Technical Report arXiv:2006.06744, arXiv, 2020.

[14] Filio Marinelli, Gregory Tsoucalas, Marianna Karaminou, and George Androutsos. Mary Mallon (1869–1938) and the history of typhoid fever. *Annals of Gastroenterology*, 26(2):123–134, 2013.

[15] Michael Molloy and Bruce Reed. A critical point for random graphs with a given degree sequence. *Random Structures and Algorithms*, 6(2–3), March–May 1995.

[16] M.E.J. Newman. *Networks: an introduction*. Oxford University Press, 2010.

[17] M.E.J. Newman, Duncan Watts, and Steven Strogatz. Random graph models of social networks. *Proceedings of the National Academy of Sciences*, 19, 2002.

[18] J.S. Oxford, A. Sefton, R. Jackson, W. Innes, R.S. Daniels, and N.P.A.S. Johnson. World War I may have allowed the emergence of the 'Spanish' influenza. *Lancet Infectious Diseases*, 2(2):111–114, February 2002.

[19] Mason Porter and James Gleeson. Dynamical systems on networks: a tutorial. Technical Report arXiv:1403.7663v1, arXiv, 2014.

[20] Carlo Rovelli. *Reality is not what it seems: The journey to quantum gravity*. Penguin, 2017.

[21] Hiroki Sayama. *Introduction to the modeling and analysis of complex systems*. SUNY Open Textbooks, 2015.

[22] Saray Shai and Simon Dobson. Coupled adaptive complex networks. *Physical Review E*, 87(4), April 2013.

[23] Barney Sloane. *The Black Death in London*. The History Press, 2011.

[24] Laura Spinney. *Pale Rider: The Spanish flu epidemic of 1918 and how it changed the world*. Vintage, 2018.

[25] Sara Toth Stub. Venice's Black Death and the dawn of quarantine. *Sapiens*, April 2020.

[26] Paul Taylor. Susceptible, infectious, recovered. *London Review of Books*, 42(9), May 2020.

[27] Emilia Vynnycky, Amy Trindall, and Punam Mangtani. Estimates of the reproduction numbers of Spanish influenza using morbidity data. *International Journal of Epidemiology*, 36:881–889, 2007.

[28] Jacco Wallinga and Marc Lipsitch. How generation intervals shape the relationship between growth rates and reproductive numbers. *Proceedings of the Royal Society B*, 274:599–604, 2007.

[29] Duncan Watts. *Small worlds*. Princeton Studies in Complexity. Princeton University Press, 1999.

[30] Duncan Watts and Steven Strogatz. Collective dynamics of 'small-world' networks. *Nature*, 393:440–442, 1998.

[31] Soon-Hyung Yook, Hawoong Jeong, and Albert-László Barabási. Modelling the Internet's large-scale topology. *Proceedings of the National Academy of Sciences*, 99(21), October 2002.

[32] Philip Ziegler. *The Black Death*. Sutton, 2003.

Index

Lightning Source UK Ltd.
Milton Keynes UK
UKHW052356230720
367054UK00003B/29